750
Questions & Answers about Acupuncture

Exam Preparation & Study Guide

By Fred Jennes

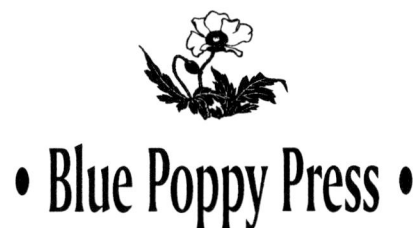

• Blue Poppy Press •

Published by:
BLUE POPPY PRESS
A Division of Blue Poppy Enterprises, Inc.
5441 Western Ave., Suite 2
BOULDER, CO 80301

First Edition, January, 2003
Second Printing, March, 2005
Third Printing, April, 2006

ISBN 1-891845-22-5
LC#2002096244

DISCLAIMER: The information in this book is given in good faith. However, the
author and the publishers cannot be held responsible for any error or omission. The
publishers will not accept liabilities for any injuries or damages caused to the reader
that may result from the reader's acting upon or using the content contained in this
book. The publishers make this information available to English language readers
for research and scholarly purposes only.

The publishers do not advocate nor endorse self-medication by laypersons. Chinese
medicine is a professional medicine. Laypersons interested in availing themselves of
the treatments described in this book should seek out a qualified professional
practitioner of Chinese medicine.

COMP Designation: Original work using a standard translational terminology

10 9 8 7 6 5 4 3

Cover & Layout by Eric J. Brearton

Printed at EB Digital, Ann Arbor, MI

Dedication

This book is dedicated to the memory of David Leaver, L.Ac., Dipl.Ac.(NCCAOM), who passed away in the dark days of September 2001. He was a gifted teacher, compassionate practitioner, avid student of TCM, and steadfast friend. We miss him.

Acknowledgements

I began this work in late spring of 2001, paused for several months in the catastrophic fall and winter of that year, and completed it a year later. I wish to acknowledge a number of people who sustained me during this project and without whose support it would never have come to fruition.

To my publishers, Bob Flaws and Honora Wolfe, whose infinite patience and support of me during this year enabled me to complete the work with minimal "noodging" and lots of understanding.

To my friends and colleagues, Christine Thomas, Bill Hamilton, Al Lamborn, Caylor Wadlington, O.M.D., and Judi Terrell, L.Ac., who provided the right words and the right acupuncture at the right time which enabled me to persevere and get the job done.

And finally to my wife and son, Helen Reed and Alex Jennes, who unstintingly gave me permission to leave them for hours and days at a time to explore the fascinating world of Chinese medicine and produce this book.

—Fred Jennes
M.Ed., L.Ac., Dipl.Ac. & C.H. (NCCAOM)

Table Of Contents

Introduction

This book is a series of questions and answers that serve as mental calisthenics to strengthen and build the Chinese medical student's knowledge base. While it makes an ideal tool for the beginning acupuncture student who needs drill and practice to prepare of the NCCAOM Board exams as well as academy proficiency tests, it is also an excellent tool for the seasoned practitioner who needs a periodic review of the basics of acupuncture.

The book is divided into five sections. Section 1, General Theory, tests the reader's academic knowledge in three areas—channel theory, point theory, and acumoxa technique. Section 2, Point Theory, examines the reader's knowledge of how the points function—both individually as well as when combined with other points. Section 3, Mixed Channels, Section 4, Point Location, assesses the reader's skill in finding the primary channel acupoints as well as the non-channel and ear acupoints. And Section 5, the Case Studies section, combines the reader's knowledge of the prior three sections and calls upon the reader to select the appropriate point prescription for a number of real-life cases.

At the end of the book is a key that provides the reader with the answers to the questions posed by each section. As any practiced student of acupuncture knows, there is not always one answer to every Chinese medical question. An examination of any of the leading textbooks of acupuncture shows that there are many differences of opinions as to the location and function of the acupoints, as well as to the appropriate prescriptions for the multitude of Chinese medical patterns of disease. To solve this problem, I selected four leading textbooks and sought consensus among them in generating questions and answers. These are Cheng's *Chinese Acupuncture and Moxibustion* (a.k.a. CAM, 1999 revised edition), Deadman and Al-Khafaji's *A Manual of Acupuncture*, O'Connor and Bensky's translation of *Acupuncture: A Comprehensive Text* (a.k.a. Shang Hai, 1981 edition), and Flaws and Finney's *Compendium of TCM Patterns and Treatments*. My hope is that by relying on both the knowledge and the wisdom of my forebears, I have produced a text which is both accurate and useful.

May your study of Chinese medicine be fruitful and stimulating. And may this text provide you with many answers and further questions into the exciting world of acupuncture.

General Theory
Channel Theory

1. Which of the following body areas would *not* be considered yang in nature?

    a. The forehead

    b. The toes

    c. The low back

    d. The lateral aspect of the elbow

Answer: _____

Source: C-16

2. Which of the following vessels corresponds to the wood phase?

    a. Foot *jue yin*

    b. Hand *jue yin*

    c. Hand *yang ming*

    d. Foot *tai yang*

Answer: _____

Source: C-21

3. The large intestine channel corresponds with which phase?

    a. Fire

    b. Earth

    c. Metal

    d. Water

Answer: _____

Source: C-21

4. The bitter flavor corresponds with which phase?

    a. Fire

    b. Wood

    c. Earth

    d. Metal

Answer: _____

Source: C-22

5. Which phase generates water?

      a. Wood

      b. Metal

      c. Fire

      d. Earth

Answer: _b_

Source: C-23

6. Earth is restrained by which phase?

      a. Fire

      b. Metal

      c. Water

      d. Wood

Answer: _d_

Source: C-23

7. If a patient comes in with a replete pattern involving the liver, according to the five phases, which channel should you use to treat it?

      a. Heart

      b. Kidney

      c. Lung

      d. Spleen

Answer: _c_

Source: C-26

8. Which of the following is not a bowel?

      a. Large intestine

      b. Small intestine

      c. Pericardium

      d. Stomach

Answer: _c_

Source: C-63, D-14

9. In Chinese medicine there are _____ primary channels.

      a. 6

      b. 12

      c. 15

      d. 24

Answer: _____

Source: C-60, D-13

10. Including the great network vessel of the spleen, there are a total of _____ network channels.

      a. 6

      b. 12

      c. 15

      d. 24

Answer: _____

Source: C-97, D-26

11. The 15 network vessels consist of:

      a. The network vessels of the 12 regular channels and those of the governing, conception, and penetrating vessels.

      b. The network vessels of the 12 regular channels and those of the governing, conception, and girdling vessels.

      c. The network vessels of the 12 regular channels, those of the governing and conception vessels, and the great network vessels of the spleen.

      d. The network vessels of the 12 regular channels, those of the governing and conception vessels, and the great network vessel of the heart.

Answer: _C___

Source: C-60-61, D-26

12. Properly name this channel: the large intestine channel of hand _____.

      a. *Tai yin*

      b. *Jue yin*

      c. *Shao yang*

      d. *Yang ming*

Answer: _D___

Source: C-60, D-14

13. Properly name this channel: the liver channel of foot _____.

    a. *Tai yin*

    b. *Jue yin*

    c. *Tai yang*

    d. *Shao yang*

Answer: _____

Source: C-60, D-14

14. Which of these channel pairs are both *tai yin*?

    a. Lung, spleen

    b. Liver, lung

    c. Kidney, urinary bladder

    d. Lung, large intestine

Answer: _____

Source: C-60, D-14

15. Which of these channel pairs are both *tai yang*?

    a. Small intestine, heart

    b. Urinary bladder, small intestine

    c. Large intestine, lung

    d. Gallbladder, urinary bladder

Answer: _____

Source: C-60, D-14

16. The general distribution of the three hand and foot yin channels on the four extremities is:

    a. *Tai yin* is lateral; *shao yin* is medial; and *jue yin* is most medial

    b. *Tai yin* is lateral; *jue yin* is medial; and *shao yin* is most medial

    c. *Shao yin* is lateral; *tai yin* is medial; and *jue yin* is most medial

    d. *Jue yin* is lateral; *shao yin* is medial; and *tai yin* is most medial

Answer: _____

Source: C-66, D-15

17. Which of the following set of channels is out of order according to the midday-midnight diurnal flow of qi in the channels?

        a. Large intestine, stomach, spleen

        b. Heart, small intestine, kidney

        c. Triple burner, gallbladder, liver

        d. Kidney, pericardium, triple burner

Answer: _____

Source: C-66, D-15

18. Using the exterior-interior method, which of these channels are paired?

        a. Pericardium, triple burner

        b. Heart, lung

        c. Gallbladder, urinary bladder

        d. Liver, stomach

Answer: _____

Source: C-66, D-15

19. Using the exterior-interior method, which of these channels are paired?

        a. Lung, small intestine

        b. Liver, spleen

        c. Gallbladder, stomach

        d. Kidney, urinary bladder

Answer: _____

Source: C-66, D-15

20. Which of the following is *not* a function of the channels and collaterals?

        a. Transporting qi and blood

        b. Regulating yin and yang

        c. Protecting the body from pathogens

        d. None of the above

Answer: _____

Source: C-61-62, D-12

21. Where do the divergent channels separate from their primary channel?

    a. At the abdomen

    b. At the head and neck

    c. At the limbs

    d. In the thoracic cavity

Answer: _____

Source: C-89, D-16

22. Which of the following is *false* regarding the channel-like sinews?

    a. They circulate qi on the periphery of the body.

    b. Each penetrates its related viscus or bowel.

    c. They all originate at the extremities.

    d. They take their names from their associated primary channel.

Answer: _____

Source: C-100, D-26

23. Which of the following statements is *true* regarding the cutaneous regions?

    a. They lie beneath the channel-like sinews.

    b. They rarely manifest a deep lying disorder.

    c. Their color is used to denote pathogen invasion or traumatic injury.

    d. For effective treatment they must be deeply needled.

Answer: _____

Source: C-112-114, D-27

24. Which of the following is *true* about the extraordinary vessels?

    a. They all connect to their own viscus or bowel.

    b. They act as reservoirs, filling and emptying in response to conditions of the regular channels.

    c. They all have unique points of their own.

    d. They all have source points.

Answer: _____

Source: C-82, D-47

25. Which of these extraordinary vessels does not share its acupuncture points with other primary channels?

    a. Yin linking

    b. Yang springing

    c. Penetrating

    d. Conception

Answer: _____

Source: C-82, D-17

26. Which point is the master point of the penetrating vessel?

    a. The uniting point of the foot *yang ming* channel

    b. The network point of the foot *tai yin* channel

    c. The network point of the hand *tai yin* channel

    d. The source point of the hand *yang ming* channel

Answer: _____

Source: C-83, D-45

27. Another name for the penetrating vessel is:

    a. The sea of blood

    b. The sea of grain

    c. The sea of qi

    d. None of the above

Answer: _____

Source: C-82, D-17

28. Which set of intersection points is associated with the yin springing vessel?

    a. *Zhao Hai* (Ki 6), *Jiao Xin* (Ki 8), *Jing Ming* (Bl 1)

    b. *Hui Yin* (CV 1), *Yin Jiao* (CV 7), *Qi Chong* (St 30), *Heng Gu* (Ki 11), *You Men* (Ki 21)

    c. *Zhu Bin* (Ki 9), *Cheng Men* (Sp 12), *Fu She* (Sp 13), *Da Heng* (Sp 15), *Fu Ai* (Sp 16), *Qi Men* (Liv 14), *Tian Tu* (CV 22), *Lian Quan* (CV 23)

    d. *Jin Men* (Bl 63), *Yang Jiao* (GB 35), *Nao Shu* (SI 10), *Tian Liao* (TB 15), *Tou Wei* (St 8), *Ben Shen* (GB 13), *Jian Jing* (GB 21), *Ya Men* (GV 15), *Feng Fu* (GV 16)

Answer: _____

Source: C-85-86, D-23

29. Which set of intersection points is associated with the girdling vessel?

    a. *Hui Yin* (CV 1), *Yin Jiao* (CV 7), *Qi Chong* (St 30), *Heng Gu* (Ki 11)-*You Men* (Ki 21)

    b. *Dai Mai* (GB 26), *Wu Shu* (GB 27), *Wei Dao* (GB 28)

    c. *Zhao Hai* (Ki 6), *Jiao Xin* (Ki 8), *Jing Ming* (Bl 1)

    d. *Shen Mai* (Bl 62), *Pu Can* (Bl 61), *Fu Yang* (Bl 59), *Ju Liao* (GB 29), *Nao Shu* (SI 10), *Jian Yu* (LI 15), *Ju Gu* (LI 16), *Di Cang* (St 4), *Ju Liao* (St 3), *Cheng Chi* (St 1), *Jing Ming* (Bl 1), *Feng Chi* (GB 20)

Answer: _____

Source: C-84,85, D-18

30. Which of the extraordinary vessels starts from the inside of the lower abdomen and emerges at the perineum?

    a. Yang springing vessel

    b. Yin springing vessel

    c. Girdling vessel

    d. Penetrating vessel

Answer: _____

Source: C-83, D-18

31. Which one of the extraordinary vessels runs posteriorly along the interior of the spinal column to the nape of the neck?

    a. Yin linking vessel

    b. Yang linking vessel

    c. Governing vessel

    d. Conception vessel

Answer: _____

Source: C-83, D-529

32. Which of the extraordinary vessels is used to treat a patient who has a "sensation at the waist as though sitting in water?"

    a. Yang springing vessel

    b. Yin linking vessel

    c. Girdling vessel

    d. Penetrating vessel

Answer: _____

Source: D-20

Sources: C=CAM, D=Deadman, F=Flaws, S=Shanghai

33. Which of the extraordinary vessels is used to treat patients with chest or heart pain?

    a. Yin springing vessel

    b. Penetrating vessel

    c. Conception vessel

    d. Yin linking vessel

Answer: _____

Source: D-22

Point Theory

34. Which of the following is *true*?

    a. The well point on a yin channel is a wood point, while the well point on a yang channel is a metal point.

    b. The well point on a yin channel is a metal point, while the well point on a yang channel is a fire point.

    c. The well point on a yin channel is a water point, while the well point on a yang channel is an earth point.

    d. The well point on a yin channel is a metal point, while the well point on a yang channel is a wood point.

Answer: _____

Source: C-384, D-29

35. Which group of points is classically used for clearing heat and draining fire from the body?

    a. Stream points

    b. Uniting points

    c. Brook points

    d. River points

Answer: _____

Source: C-382, D-33

36. The deepest of the five transport points are the:

    a. Brook points

    b. Well points

    c. Stream points

    d. Uniting points

Answer: _____

Source: C-122, D-31

37. According to the *Classic of Difficulties*, the stream points are best for:

  a. Heat in the body

  b. Heaviness of the body and joint pain

  c. Fullness below the heart

  d. Counterflow qi

Answer: _____

Source: D-31, 34

38. According to the *Spiritual Pivot*, when the disease is at the sinews and bones, needle the _____ on the yin channels.

  a. Stream points

  b. Uniting points

  c. Well points

  d. River points

Answer: _____

Source: D-31, 35

39. According to the *Spiritual Pivot*, diseases of the spleen and stomach caused by irregular eating and drinking are best treated by the:

  a. Uniting points

  b. Stream points

  c. River points

  d. Brook points

Answer: _____

Source: D-31, 36

40. Well points:

  a. Are located near knees and elbows

  b. Are always associated with metal phase

  c. Are able to treat severe febrile illnesses

  d. Are source points on the yin channels

Answer: _____

Source: C-382, D-32

41. According to the *Classic of Difficulties*, "In cases of vacuity, supplement the _____; in cases of repletion drain the _____."

    a. Child, mother

    b. Mother, child

    c. Child, grandparent

    d. Grandparent, mother

Answer: _____

Source: D-37

42. In the five phase system, on a yin channel, the well point is always the _____ phase.

    a. Metal

    b. Water

    c. Wood

    d. Fire

Answer: _____

Source: D-37

43. Cleft points are generally used to treat what kind of conditions?

    a. Damp

    b. Acute

    c. Chronic

    d. Resolving

Answer: _____

Source: C-125, D-38

44. On yin channels, the stream point is also the _____ point.

    a. Network

    b. Cleft

    c. Back transport

    d. Source

Answer: _____

Source: C-123, D-39

45. According to the *Guide to the Classic of Acupuncture*, the network points should be paired with the _____ points of their interiorly-exteriorly related channel.

    a. Cleft

    b. Uniting

    c. Source

    d. Back transport

Answer: _____

Source: D-41

46. According to the *Spiritual Pivot*, back transport points are located:

    a. Above their corresponding viscus or bowel

    b. Below their corresponding viscus or bowel

    c. By palpating for tenderness or soreness

    d. On the abdomen

Answer: _____

Source: C-123, D-43

47. The alarm points are located:

    a. On the chest or abdomen

    b. Near their respective back transport points

    c. Along the limbs

    d. By palpating the spine

Answer: _____

Source: D-43-44

48. Which is *true* of back transport points?

    a. They are found on each of the 12 regular channels.

    b. They are all found on the eight extraordinary vessels.

    c. They are all found on the bladder channel.

    d. They are all found on the legs.

Answer: _____

Source: C-392, D-42

49. According to the *Classic of Difficulties*, which of these is *not* a master point?

    a. Viscera

    b. Bowels

    c. Blood

    d. Yin

Answer: _____

Source: C-124, D-44

50. In the *Glorious Anthology of Acupuncture and Moxibustion*, four command points were identified. Respectively these treated the abdomen, lumbar region, face and mouth, and:

    a. Limbs

    b. Viscera

    c. Bowels

    d. Nape of the neck

Answer: _____

Source: D-47

51. The *Spiritual Pivot* identified four sea points. Which of the following is *not* one of these four points?

    a. Sea of grain

    b. Sea of spirit

    c. Sea of blood

    d. Sea of marrow

Answer: _____

Source: D-47, 48

52. The *Spiritual Pivot* first identified a group of 10 points called "heavenly window" points, because they have *tian* in their name. With two exceptions, these points are generally found:

    a. On the legs

    b. Along the spine

    c. On the belly

    d. Around the head and neck

Answer: _____

Source: D-48, 49

53. Which of these disorders is *not* generally treated by heavenly window points?

     a. Sudden onset disorders

     b. Mental and emotional disorders

     c. Musculoskeletal disorders

     d. Sense organ disorders

Answer: _____

Source: D-49, 50

54. In the *Essential Formulas [Worth] a Thousand [Pieces of] Gold,* Sun Si-Mao identified 13 points for the treatment of manias and epilepsy. These are called:

     a. Curative points

     b. Heavenly spirit points

     c. Ghost points

     d. Spirit restorative points

Answer: _____

Source: D-50, 51

55. Which of the following points intersects the three foot yin vessels plus the conception vessel?

     a. *San Yin Jiao* (Sp 6)

     b. *Bing Fang* (SI 12)

     c. *Da Zhui* (GV 14)

     d. *Zhong Ji* (CV 3)

Answer: _____

Source: C-397, D-55

56. At which point do all the yang vessels cross?

     a. *Jing Ming* (Bl 1)

     b. *Bai Hui* (GV 20)

     c. *Da Zhui* (GV 14)

     d. *Bing Fang* (SI 12)

Answer: _____

Source: C-394, D-54

Technique

57. The distance from the anterior to posterior hairline is:

    a. 8 *cun*

    b. 9 *cun*

    c. 12 *cun*

    d. 13 *cun*

Answer: _____

Source: C-119, D-63

58. The distance between the transverse cubital crease and the transverse wrist crease is:

    a. 9 *cun*

    b. 12 *cun*

    c. 13 *cun*

    d. 16 *cun*

Answer: _____

Source: C-120, D-63

59. The distance between the prominence of the great trochanter to the middle of the patella is:

    a. 12 *cun*

    b. 16 *cun*

    c. 18 *cun*

    d. 19 *cun*

Answer: _____

Source: C-120, D-64

60. The distance between the two nipples is:

    a. 4 *cun*

    b. 6 *cun*

    c. 8 *cun*

    d. 9 *cun*

Answer: _____

Source: C-119, D-63

61. The distance between the sternocostal angle to the center of the umbilicus is:

    a. *5 cun*

    b. *8 cun*

    c. *9 cun*

    d. *12 cun*

Answer: _____

Source: C-119, D-63

62. Which of the following equals 16 *cun*?

    a. Cubital crease to the wrist crease

    b. Lateral malleolus to the femur head

    c. Lateral malleolus to the center of the patella

    d. Xiphoid process to the superior border of the pubic bone

Answer: _____

Source: C-119, 120, D-63, 64

63. What is the distance from the end of the axillary fold to the wrist crease?

    a. 12 *cun*

    b. 21 *cun*

    c. 9 *cun*

    d. 18 *cun*

Answer: _____

Source: C-120, D-63

64. The distance from the midline of the sternum to the mammillary line is:

    a. 8 *cun*

    b. 4 *cun*

    c. 6 *cun*

    d. 2 *cun*

Answer: _____

Source: C-118, D-63

65. The distance from the umbilicus to the superior border of the pubic bone is:

    a. 8 *cun*

    b. 4 *cun*

    c. 5 *cun*

    d. 2 *cun*

Answer: _____

Source: C-119, D-64

66. The demarcation line between the body and handle of the filiform needle is called the:

    a. Tip

    b. Tail

    c. Root

    d. Union

Answer: _____

Source: C-337

67. Which of the following filiform needle measurements has the smallest diameter?

    a. 40 gauge

    b. 36 gauge

    d. 34 gauge

    d. Cannot be determined from this information

Answer: _____

Source: C-338

68. A filiform needle insertion at an angle of 45° is called a(n) _____ insertion.

    a. Perpendicular

    b. Oblique

    c. Transverse

    d. Horizontal

Answer: _____

Source: C-343, D-65

69. A horizontal insertion is usually used:

    a. In the buttocks

    b. On the extremities

    c. On the head or forehead   ✓

    d. On the abdomen

Answer: _____

Source: C-343

70. Which of the following needling techniques is used for draining?

    a. Plucking

    b. Scraping

    c. Shaking ✓

    d. Flying

Answer: _____

Source: C-344

71. Which of the following needling techniques is *not* used for supplementing?

    a. Inserting the needle in the direction in which the channel runs.

    b. Inserting the needle when the patient breathes in.

    c. Pressing the hole on withdrawal of the needle.

    d. All of the above are supplementing needling techniques.

Answer: _____

Source: C-348, 349

72. For which of the following conditions is using a three-edged needle to bleed an acupoint inappropriate?

    a. Blood stasis

    b. Qi and blood vacuity ✓

    c. Sore throat from wind heat

    d. All of the above

Answer: _____

Source: C-354

Sources: C=CAM, D=Deadman, F=Flaws, S=Shanghai

73. Seven star or plum blossom needles can be used to treat:

    a. Nervous system disorders

    b. Skin diseases

    c. Dizziness and vertigo

    d. All of the above

Answer: _____

Source: C-355

74. What is the chief precaution associated with intradermal needles?

    a. The patient can become dizzy if they are put in the ear.

    b. The needle site can become infected, especially in summer.

    c. They should not be used on women with menstrual disorders.

    d. They should not be used with chronic or painful conditions.

Answer: _____

Source: C-356

75. Which of these is *not* a function of moxa?

    a. Regulating the qi and blood

    b. Expelling cold from the vessels

    c. Resolving dampness

    d. Supplementing yin

Answer: _____

Source: C-361

76. When employing indirect moxa, which of the following substances is the most effective for treating a vacuity of lifegate fire?

    a. Fresh ginger

    b. Garlic

    c. Aconite

    d. Salt

Answer: _____

Source: C-365

77. For which of these conditions is moxa appropriate?

    a. When the patient has a high fever to drain it with fire.

    b. On the abdomen of a pregnant woman to give the fetus more yang qi.

    c. Near *Jing Ming* (Bl 1) to increase the brightness in the eyes when the patient has cataracts.

    d. Moxa should not be used in any of the above conditions.

Answer: _____

Source: C-368

78. Which of the following conditions would *not* be an appropriate condition for treatment with cups?

    a. Bleeding disorders due to blood vacuity

    b. Lung disorders, especially from wind evils

    c. Low back pain from trauma

    d. All of the above conditions are appropriate conditions for cupping

Answer: _____

Source: C-369

Point Theory
Lung

79. Identify the uniting point on the lung channel.

      a. *Chi Ze* (Lu 5)

      b. *Lie Que* (Lu 7)

      c. *Tai Yuan* (Lu 9)

      d. *Shao Shang* (Lu 11)

Answer: _____

Source: C-136, D-80

80. Which acupoint is best for supplementing the lungs?

      a. *Chi Ze* (Lu 5)

      b. *Lie Que* (Lu 7)

      c. *Jing Gu* (Lu 8)

      d. *Tai Yuan* (Lu 9)

Answer: _____

Source: C-138, D-86

81. Identify the cleft point on the lung channel.

      a. *Kong Zui* (Lu 6)

      b. *Lie Que* (Lu 7)

      c. *Jing Qu* (Lu 8)

      d. *Yu Ji* (Lu 10)

Answer: _____

Source: C-137, D-82

82. Which acupoint on the lung channel is also the master point of an extraordinary vessel?

    a. *Zhong Fu* (Lu 1)

    b. *Chi Ze* (Lu 5)

    c. *Lie Que* (Lu 7)

    d. *Jing Qu* (Lu 8)

Answer: _____

Source: C-137, D-83

83. Which acupoint on the lung channel is the fire point?

    a. *Chi Ze* (Lu 5)

    b. *Kong Zui* (Lu 6)

    c. *Jing Qu* (Lu 8)

    d. *Yu Ji* (Lu 10)

Answer: _____

Source: C-138, D-88

84. What is the child point on the lung channel?

    a. *Zhong Fu* (Lu 1)

    b. *Chi Ze* (Lu 5)

    c. *Jing Qu* (Lu 8)

    d. *Shao Shang* (Lu 11)

Answer: _____

Source: C-136, D-80

85. In the event of an acute repletion pattern involving phlegm in the lungs, which would be the best point to choose?

    a. The alarm point

    b. The uniting point

    c. The cleft point

    d. The source point

Answer: _____

Source: C-137, D-82

86. Which acupoint would be best selected for treating lung qi and yin vacuity?

    a. *Zhong Fu* (Lu 1)

    b. *Kong Zhi* (Lu 6)

    c. *Jing Qu* (Lu 8)

    d. *Shao Shang* (Lu 11)

Answer: _____

Source: F-102, D-76

87. How many acupoints are on the lung channel?

    a. 9

    b. 10

    c. 11

    d. 20

Answer: _____

Source: C-135, D-73

88. For wind cold raiding the lungs, the primary acupoint on the lung channel to choose would be:

    a. The uniting point

    b. The cleft point

    c. The network point

    d. The river point

Answer: _____

Source: F-85, D-83

89. For a severe sore throat as the result of wind heat attacking the lungs, you would bleed:

    a. *Zhong Fu* (Lu 1)

    b. *Lie Que* (Lu 7)

    c. *Jing Qu* (Lu 8)

    d. *Shao Shang* (Lu 11)

Answer: _____

Source: F-86, D-90

90. Which acupoint on the lung channel corresponds to the metal phase?

     a. *Tai Yuan* (Lu 9)

     b. *Jing Qu* (Lu 8)

     c. *Chi Ze* (Lu 5)

     d. *Zhong Fu* (Lu 1)

Answer: _____

Source: C-138, D-86

91. Identify the source point on the lung channel.

     a. *Zhong Fu* (Lu 1)

     b. *Chi Ze* (Lu 5)

     c. *Jing Qu* (Lu 8)

     d. *Tai Yuan* (Lu 9)

Answer: _____

Source: C-138, D-86

92. The uniting point on the lung is also called the _____ point.

     a. Water

     b. Well

     c. Cleft

     d. Alarm

Answer: _____

Source: C-136, D-80

Large Intestine

93. Which of the following is the correct name for the large intestine channel?

    a. Foot *yang ming*

    b. Hand *yang ming*

    c. Hand *tai yin*

    d. Foot *shao yang*

Answer: _____

Source: C-139, D-95

94. What is the network point on the large intestine channel?

    a. *Shang Yang* (LI 1)

    b. *He Gu* (LI 4)

    c. *Yang Xi* (LI 5)

    d. *Pian Li* (LI 6)

Answer: _____

Source: C-141, D-108

95. What is the primary function of *Jian Yu* (LI 15)?

    a. Treating invasion of wind evils

    b. Treating anterior shoulder pain

    c. Treating posterior shoulder pain

    d. Treating heat in the *yang ming* channels

Answer: _____

Source: C-142, D-112

96. Which acupoint on the large intestine channel corresponds to the wood phase?

    a. *Er Jian* (LI 2)

    b. *San Jian* (LI 3)

    c. *He Gu* (LI 4)

    d. *Qu Chi* (LI 11)

Answer: _____

Source: C-384, D-102

97. This acupoint, which treats a large number of conditions involving the nose, is also an intersection point of the hand and foot *yang ming* channels:

    a. *He Gu* (LI 4)

    b. *Wen Liu* (LI 7)

    c. *Kou He Liao* (LI 19)

    d. *Ying Xiang* (LI 20)

Answer: _____

Source: C-144, D-116

98. What is the grandparent point on the large intestine channel?

    a. The well point

    b. The brook point

    c. The river point

    d. The uniting point

Answer: _____

Source: C-384, D-37

99. Which point on the large intestine channel is the most effective for treating damp heat causing abdominal pain and diarrhea?

    a. *Shang Yang* (LI 1)

    b. *Er Jian* (LI 2)

    c. *Wen Liu* (LI 7)

    d. *Qu Chi* (LI 11)

Answer: _____

Source: C-142, D-112, F-112

100. What is the source point on the large intestine channel?

    a. *Shang Yang* (LI 1)

    b. *He Gu* (LI 4)

    c. *Yang Xi* (LI 5)

    d. *Qu Chi* (LI 11)

Answer: _____

Source: C-140, D-103

101. How many points are on the large intestine channel?

    a. 11

    b. 15

    c. 20

    d. 23

Answer: _____

Source: C-144, D-120

102. For wind heat attacking the lungs, in addition to *Qu Chi* (LI 11), the best point for treating the patient would be:

    a. *Shang Yang* (LI 2)

    b. *San Jian* (LI 3)

    c. *He Gu* (LI 4)

    d. *Wen Liu* (LI 7)

Answer: _____

Source: C-140, D-103, F-85

103. What is the lower uniting point of the large intestine channel?

    a. *He Gu* (LI 4)

    b. *Qu Chi* (LI 11)

    c. *Jian Yu* (LI 15)

    d. *Shang Ju Xu* (St 37)

Answer: _____

Source: C-154, D-162

104. To drain the large intestine channel, the best point to choose would be:

    a. The well point

    b. The brook point

    c. The source point

    d. The cleft point

Answer: _____

Source: C-385, D-101

105. Identify the alarm point of the large intestine channel.

     a. *He Gu* (LI 4)

     b. *Tian Shu* (St 25)

     c. *Zu San Li* (St 36)

     d. *Zhong Wan* (CV 12)

Answer: _____

Source: C-151, D-148

106. Which point on the large intestine channel is a command point effective for treating epistaxis?

     a. *He Gu* (LI 4)

     b. *Qu Chi* (LI 11)

     c. *Bi Nao* (LI 14)

     d. *Ying Xiang* (LI 20)

Answer: _____

Source: C-382, D-47

Stomach

107. Which point on the stomach channel is the command point for disorders of the abdomen?

    a. *Tian Shu* (St 25)

    b. *Qi Chong* (St 30)

    c. *Zu San Li* (St 36)

    d. *Chong Yang* (St 42)

Answer: _____

Source: C-382, D-47

108. Identify the cleft point on the stomach channel:

    a. *Qi Chong* (St 30)

    b. *Liang Qiu* (St 34)

    c. *Zu San Li* (St 36)

    d. *Feng Long* (St 40)

Answer: _____

Source: C-156, D-168

109. What is the primary function of *Tiao Kou* (St 38)?

    a. Prevents wind invasion of the stomach

    b. Treats pain and motor impairment of the shoulder

    c. Improves digestion

    d. Stops epistaxis

Answer: _____

Source: C-155, D-163

110. The uniting point on the stomach channel is also the _____ point.

    a. River

    b. Earth

    c. Cleft

    d. Alarm

Answer: _____

Source: C-154, D-158

111. Which acupoint on the stomach channel is the lower uniting point of the small intestine channel?

    a. *Zu San Li* (St 36)

    b. *Shang Ju Xu* (St 37)

    c. *Xia Ju Xu* (St 39)

    d. *Xiang Gu* (St 43)

Answer: _____

Source: C-155, D-164

112. This acupoint on the stomach channel is the "calf's nose" which treats knee pain:

    a. *Liang Qiu* (St 34)

    b. *Du Bi* (St 35)

    c. *Zu San Li* (St 36)

    d. *Feng Long* (St 40)

Answer: _____

Source: C-154, D-157

113. Identify the river point on the stomach channel.

    a. *Jie Xi* (St 41)

    b. *Chong Yang* (St 42)

    c. *Xiang Gu* (St 43)

    d. *Nei Ting* (St 44)

Answer: _____

Source: C-155, D-167

114. In addition to *Ru Gen* (St 18), which acupoint on the stomach channel can be needled to treat mastitis?

    a. *Ru Zhong* (St 17)

    b. *Cheng Man* (St 20)

    c. *Liang Qiu* (St 34)

    d. *Li Dui* (St 45)

Answer: _____

Source: C-154, D-156

115. Which acupoint on the stomach channel treats most nasal problems, including swelling and epistaxis?

      a. *Ju Liao* (St 3)

      b. *Di Cang* (St 4)

      c. *Da Ying* (St 5)

      d. *Jia Che* (St 6)

Answer: _____

Source: C-145, D-131

116. Name the alarm point of the stomach channel.

      a. *Tian Shu* (St 25)

      b. *Zu San Li* (St 36)

      c. *Zhong Wan* (CV 12)

      d. *Tan Zhong* (CV 17)

Answer: _____

Source: C-238, D-511

117. Identify the network point on the stomach channel.

      a. *Liang Qiu* (St 34)

      b. *Zu San Li* (St 36)

      c. *Shang Ju Xu* (St 37)

      d. *Feng Long* (St 40)

Answer: _____

Source: C-155, D-165

118. For stomach fire hyperactivity patterns due to eating acrid, hot, peppery foods, which key point on the stomach channel should be supplemented to quell the problem?

      a. *Liang Qiu* (St 34)

      b. *Zu San Li* (St 36)

      c. *Shang Ju Xu* (St 37)

      d. *Nei Ting* (St 44)

Answer: _____

Source: C-156, D-171, F-78

119. What is the upper sea point of water and grain?

    a. *Qi Chong* (St 30)

    b. *Zu San Li* (St 36)

    c. *Shang Ju Xu* (St 37)

    d. *Xia Ju Xu* (St 39)

Answer: _____

Source: C-152, D-152

120. What is the primary function of *Fu Tu* (St 32)?

    a. To treat acute gastritis

    b. To regulate menstruation

    c. To dispel cold and damp from the lower limbs

    d. To clear heat from the stomach channel

Answer: _____

Source: C-153, D-155

121. Which acupoint on the stomach channel has the function of transforming and clearing phlegm anywhere in the body?

    a. The well point

    b. The earth point

    c. The water point

    d. The network point

Answer: _____

Source: C-155, D-165

122. The stomach channel point best known for dispersing swelling is:

    a. The uniting point

    b. The stream point

    c. The metal point

    d. The source point

Answer: _____

Source: C-156, D-170

123. Which point on the stomach channel is the upper point of the sea of qi?

        a. *Jia Che* (St 6)

        b. *Ren Ying* (St 9)

        c. *Tian Shu* (St 25)

        d. *Zu San Li* (St 36)

Answer: _____

Source: C-147, D-137

124. This acupoint on the stomach channel is one of the most important for treating headaches of any etiology:

        a. *Cheng Qi* (St 1)

        b. *Di Cang* (St 4)

        c. *Jia Che* (St 6)

        d. *Tou Wei* (St 8)

Answer: _____

Source: C-147, D-135

125. Which point on the stomach channel is key for treating most patterns involving the jaw?

        a. *Jia Che* (St 6)

        b. *Xia Guan* (St 7)

        c. *Liang Qiu* (St 34)

        d. *Zu San Li* (St 36)

Answer: _____

Source: C-146, D-133

Sources: C=CAM, D=Deadman, F=Flaws, S=Shanghai

Spleen

126. How many acupoints are on the spleen channel?

    a. 9

    b. 20

    c. 21

    d. 23

Answer: _____

Source: C-157, D-177

127. The spleen channel has two network points. One is *Gong Sun* (Sp 4), the other is _____.

    a. *San Yin Jiao* (Sp 6)

    b. *Xue Hai* (Sp 10)

    c. *Da Heng* (Sp 15)

    d. *Da Bao* (Sp 21)

Answer: _____

Source: C-204, D-163

128. Which acupoint on the spleen channel corresponds to the water phase?

    a. *Yin Ling Quan* (Sp 9)

    b. *San Yin Jiao* (Sp 6)

    c. *Shang Qiu* (Sp 5)

    d. *Tai Bai* (Sp 3)

Answer: _____

Source: C-159, D-194

129. This acupoint, often referred to as the "cleft point of blood," is key for regulating menstruation:

    a. *Tai Bai* (Sp 3)

    b. *San Yin Jiao* (Sp 6)

    c. *Di Ji* (Sp 8)

    d. *Xue Hai* (Sp 10)

Answer: _____

Source: C-159, D-193

130. Which point on the spleen channel is a master point of an extraordinary vessel?

      a. *Da Bao* (Sp 21)

      b. *Xue Hai* (Sp 10)

      c. *San Yin Jiao* (Sp 6)

      d. *Gong Sun* (Sp 4)

Answer: _____

Source: C-158, D-186

131. Identify the brook point on the spleen channel.

      a. *Lou Gu* (Sp 7)

      b. *Shang Qiu* (Sp 5)

      c. *Gong Sun* (Sp 4)

      d. *Da Du* (Sp 2)

Answer: _____

Source: C-157, D-183

132. Which point on the spleen channel is the intersection point of the three foot yin channels?

      a. *Tai Bai* (Sp 3)

      b. *San Yin Jiao* (Sp 6)

      c. *Yin Ling Quan* (Sp 9)

      d. *Da Bao* (Sp 21)

Answer: _____

Source: C-158, D-189

133. In addition to quickening the blood, *Xue Hai* (Sp 10) also:

      a. Brightens the eyes

      b. Improves digestion

      c. Treats skin rashes

      d. Resolves leg pain

Answer: _____

Source: C-160, D-196

134. The primary function of *Yin Ling Quan* (Sp 9) is to treat:

    a. Menstrual disorders due to blood stasis

    b. Leg pain due to trauma

    c. Urinary dysfunctions due to heat conditions

    d. Abdominal pain and distention due to damp conditions

Answer: _____

Source: C-159, D-194

135. Which point on the spleen channel is bled to stop menorrhagia?

    a. The well point

    b. The network point

    c. The cleft point

    d. The source point

Answer: _____

Source: C-157, D-182

136. What is the alarm point of the spleen channel?

    a. *Da Heng* (Sp 15)

    b. *Da Bao* (Sp 21)

    c. *Zhang Men* (Liv 13)

    d. Zhong Wan (CV 12)

Answer: _____

Source: C-226, D-488

137. The source point on the spleen channel is also the _____ point.

    a. Metal

    b. Earth

    c. Wood

    d. Fire

Answer: _____

Source: C-384, D-184

138. Which acupoint on the spleen channel is the mother point?

    a. The fire point

    b. The stream point

    c. The cleft point

    d. The network point

Answer: _____

Source: C-385, D-37

139. Which point on the spleen channel is best for treating general achiness or weakness of the entire body?

    a. *Tai Bai* (Sp 3)

    b. *Gong Sun* (Sp 4)

    c. *Di Ji* (Sp 8)

    d. *Da Bao* (Sp 21)

Answer: _____

Source: C-163, D-204

Heart

140. Which of the following is the correct name for the heart channel?

    a. Hand *tai yang*

    b. Hand *shao yin*

    c. Hand *jue yin*

    d. Hand *tai yin*

Answer: _____

Source: C-164, D-209

141. Which acupoint on the heart channel is the water point?

    a. The uniting point

    b. The stream point

    c. The cleft point

    d. The source point

Answer: _____

Source: C-384, D-214

142. Identify the alarm point of the heart channel.

    a. *Shen Men* (Ht 7)

    b. *Ju Que* (CV 14)

    c. *Jiu Wei* (CV 15)

    d. *Tan Zhong* (CV 17)

Answer: _____

Source: C-239, D-514

143. To drain the heart, the best point on the heart channel is:

    a. The fire point

    b. The cleft point

    c. The source point

    d. The river point

Answer: _____

Source: C-166, D-219

144. The best point on the heart channel for treating sudden loss of voice or aphasia is:

    a. *Tong Li* (Ht 5)

    b. *Yin Xi* (Ht 6)

    c. *Shao Fu* (Ht 8)

    d. *Shen Men* (Ht 9)

Answer: _____

Source: C-165, D-216

145. Which of the following statements is *false*?

    a. The fire point on the heart channel is also the horary point.

    b. The horary point on the heart channel is also the brook point.

    c. The fire point on the heart channel is also the draining point.

    d. The horary point on the heart channel is *Shao Fu* (Ht 8).

Answer: _____

Source: C-166, D-221

146. Which acupoint on the heart channel is best for treating either vacuity or repletion patterns of insomnia?

    a. *Ji Quan* (Ht 1)

    b. *Tong Li* (Ht 5)

    c. *Shen Men* (Ht 7)

    d. *Shao Chong* (Ht 9)

Answer: _____

Source: C-166, D-219

147. Which acupoint on the heart channel should be bled for loss of consciousness?

    a. *Ji Quan* (Ht 1)

    b. *Shen Men* (Ht 7)

    c. *Shao Fu* (Ht 8)

    d. *Shao Chong* (Ht 9)

Answer: _____

Source: C-166, D-222

148. What is the grandparent point on the heart?

    a. *Shao Hai* (Ht 3)

    b. *Ling Dao* (Ht 4)

    c. *Shen Men* (Ht 7)

    d. *Shao Chong* (Ht 9)

Answer: _____

Source: C-166, D-214

Small Intestine

149. How many points are on the small intestine channel?

    a. 19

    b. 20

    c. 21

    d. 23

Answer: _____

Source: C-173, D-247

150. Which acupoint on the small intestine channel corresponds to the earth phase?

    a. The well point

    b. The source point

    c. The child point

    d. The supplementation point

Answer: _____

Source: C-384, D-29

151. What is the empirical use of the source point on the small intestine channel?

    a. It treats eye pain.

    b. It treats low back pain.

    c. It treats pain in the calf.

    d. It treats jaundice.

Answer: _____

Source: C-168, D-235

152. Identify the supplementation point on the small intestine channel.

    a. *Shao Ze* (SI 1)

    b. *Qiang Gu* (SI 2)

    c. *Hou Xi* (SI 3)

    d. *Yang Gu* (SI 5)

Answer: _____

Source: C-385, D-37

153. For a pattern of small intestine vacuity cold, one would use the lower uniting point of the small intestine, which is:

      a. *Xiao Hai* (SI 8)

      b. The fire point on the small intestine channel

      c. *Shang Ju Xiu* (St 37)

      d. *Xia Ju Xiu* (St 39)

Answer: _____

Source: C-155, D-164, F-56

154. Which of the following channels does *not* intersect at *Bing Feng* (SI 12)?

      a. The hand *tai yang*

      b. The foot *tai yang*

      c. The hand *yang ming*

      d. The hand *shao yang*

Answer: _____

Source: C-395, D-242

155. Which of the acupoints on the small intestine channel has been shown by empirical use to be effective in treating insufficient lactation?

      a. *Shao Ze* (SI 1)

      b. *Hou Xi* (SI 3)

      c. *Wan Gu* (SI 4)

      d. *Nao Shu* (SI 10)

Answer: _____

Source: C-167, D-231

156. For blurred vision involving a vacuity pattern in elderly patients, which acupoint on the small intestine channel is the best choice?

      a. *Hou Xi* (SI 3)

      b. *Wan Gu* (SI 4)

      c. *Yang Lao* (SI 6)

      d. *Xiao Hai* (SI 8)

Answer: _____

Source: C-168, D-237

157. For pain in the scapula, which local point is the best choice?

    a. *Hou Xi* (SI 3)

    b. *Yang Lao* (SI 6)

    c. *Xiao Hai* (SI 8)

    d. *Tian Zong* (SI 11)

Answer: _____

Source: C-171, D-241

158. What is the major function of *Ting Gong* (SI 19)?

    a. Treats shoulder pain

    b. Treats skin diseases

    c. Treats hearing problems

    d. Treats bladder infections

Answer: _____

Source: C-173, D-247

159. What is the alarm point of the small intestine channel?

    a. *Hou Xi* (SI 3)

    b. *Wan Gu* (SI 4)

    c. *Zhong Ji* (CV 3)

    d. *Guan Yuan* (CV 4)

Answer: _____

Source: C-237, D-501

160. Which acupoint on the small intestine channel is the master point of an extraordinary vessel?

    a. The source point

    b. The wood point

    c. The restraining point

    d. The uniting point

Answer: _____

Source: C-167, D-233

161. For severe, acute lumbar sprain which acupoint on the small intestine channel is the best choice?

     a. *Shao Ze* (SI 1)

     b. *Hou Xi* (SI 3)

     c. *Wan Gu* (SI 4)

     d. *Yang Lao* (SI 6)

Answer: _____

Source: C-168, D-237

162. Identify the network point on the small intestine channel.

     a. *Yang Gu* (SI 5)

     b. *Yang Lao* (SI 6)

     c. *Zhi Zheng* (SI 7)

     d. *Xiao Hai* (SI 8)

Answer: _____

Source: C-168, D-238

163. Which of the following statements is *true* concerning *Shao Ze* (SI 1)?

     a. It should not be used in patterns involving heat.

     b. It should only be used in vacuity patterns.

     c. It is effective for treating headaches, especially replete ones.

     d. It is the wood phase point.

Answer: _____

Source: C-167, D-231

Bladder

164. How many points are there on the bladder channel?

     a. 60

     b. 63

     c. 65

     d. 67

Answer: _____

Source: C-191, D-326

165. The bladder channel is also called:

     a. Foot *tai yang*

     b. Foot *yang ming*

     c. Foot *shao yang*

     d. Hand *tai yang*

Answer: _____

Source: C-173, D-251

166. Identify the metal phase point on the bladder channel.

     a. *Wei Zhong* (Bl 40)

     b. *Kun Lun* (Bl 60)

     c. *Jing Gu* (Bl 64)

     d. *Zhi Yin* (Bl 67)

Answer: _____

Source: C-384, D-325

167. Which of the following statements about *Jing Ming* (Bl 1) is *true*?

     a. It is the well point of the bladder channel.

     b. It treats most diseases involving the eye.

     c. It should not be needled during the last trimester of pregnancy.

     d. It should not be needled at all, only moxaed.

Answer: _____

Source: C-173, D-256

168. The bladder channel has two cleft points. One is *Jin Men* (Bl 63); what is the other?

    a. *Fei Yang* (Bl 58)

    b. *Fu Yang* (Bl 59)

    c. The river point

    d. The water point

Answer: _____

Source: C-189, D-317

169. Identify the back transport point of the pericardium channel.

    a. *Fei Shu* (Bl 13)

    b. *Jue Yin Shu* (Bl 14)

    c. *Xin Shu* (Bl 15)

    d. *Du Shu* (Bl 16)

Answer: _____

Source: C-177, D-269

170. The bladder channel has two master points. One is *Ge Shu* (Bl 17); the other is _____.

    a. The source point

    b. The network point

    c. *Da Zhu* (Bl 11)

    d. The back transport of the spleen

Answer: _____

Source: C-176, D-264

171. What is the primary function of *Feng Men* (Bl 12)?

    a. Clears the eyes

    b. Harmonizes the stomach

    c. Treats liver pattern headaches

    d. Courses wind and dispels externally contracted evils

Answer: _____

Source: C-176, D-266

172. Which acupoint on the bladder channel is the master point of an extraordinary vessel?

    a. The source point

    b. The fire point

    c. The supplementing point

    d. None of the above

Answer: _____

Source: C-320, D-190

173. Which point on the bladder channel is effective for correcting the malposition of the fetus?

    a. *Wei Zhong* (Bl 40)

    b. *Cheng Shan* (Bl 57)

    c. *Shen Mai* (Bl 62)

    d. *Zhi Yin* (Bl 67)

Answer: _____

Source: C-191, D-325

174. The bladder channel has two uniting points. One of them is *Wei Zhong* (Bl 40). Identify the other.

    a. *Fu Xi* (Bl 38)

    b. *Wei Yang* (Bl 39)

    c. *Fu Fen* (Bl 41)

    d. *Fei Yang* (Bl 58)

Answer: _____

Source: C-184, D-298

175. To treat a pattern of urinary bladder damp heat, one might use the back transport point of the bladder. Identify this acupoint.

    a. *Fei Shu* (Bl 13)

    b. *Gan Shu* (Bl 18)

    c. *Pi Shu* (Bl 20)

    d. *Pang Guang Shu* (Bl 28)

Answer: _____

Source: C-181, D-290, F-134

176. In addition to using the back transport point to treat urinary bladder damp heat, which of these alarm points would be most effective?

      a. *Zhong Ji* (CV 3)

      b. *Shi Men* (CV 5)

      c. *Zhong Wan* (CV 12)

      d. *Qi Men* (Liv 14)

Answer: _____

Source: C-499, D-136, F-134

177. Identify the network point on the bladder channel.

      a. *Shu Gu* (Bl 65)

      b. *Jing Gu* (Bl 64)

      c. *Fei Yang* (Bl 58)

      d. *Cheng Shan* (Bl 57)

Answer: _____

Source: C-188, D-316

178. Which of the following statements is false regarding the eight *liao* acupoints (Bl 31-34)?

      a. They all treat menstrual irregularities.

      b. They all treat mid-back pain.

      c. They all treat dysuria.

      d. They all treat difficulty in defecation.

Answer: _____

Source: C-182-183, D-292-295

179. To invigorate the kidneys, which back transport point should be used with needle moxa?

      a. *Xin Shu* (Bl 15)

      b. *Pi Shu* (Bl 20)

      c. *Shen Shu* (Bl 23)

      d. *Da Chang Shu* (Bl 25)

Answer: _____

Source: C-180, D-283

180. *Xiao Chang Shu* (Bl 27) is best for the treatment of:

    a. Diarrhea, especially dysentery

    b. Leg pain, especially calf cramps

    c. Low back pain, especially replete type

    d. Lung infection, especially from external evils

Answer: _____

Source: C-181, D-288

181. Which of the following statements about *Gao Huang Shu* (Bl 43) is *true*?

    a. This acupoint is best for replete patterns.

    b. This acupoint is best for vacuity patterns.

    c. This acupoint resolves damp conditions.

    d. This acupoint relieves blood stasis conditions.

Answer: _____

Source: C-185, D-304

182. Which transport point on the bladder channel is contraindicated in the first two trimesters of pregnancy?

    a. The spring point

    b. The stream point

    c. The river point

    d. The uniting point

Answer: _____

Source: C-189, D-318

183. What is the primary function of the source point on the bladder channel?

    a. Promotes urination

    b. Stops diarrhea

    c. Resolves ankle pain

    d. Clears wind from the head and neck

Answer: _____

Source: C-190, D-323

Kidney

184. Which point on the kidney channel has the primary function of regulating menstruation?

    a. The source point

    b. The cleft point

    c. The water point

    d. The fire point

Answer: _____

Source: C-193, D-343

185. The kidney channel has three cleft points. Which of these is the cleft point of the yin springing vessel?

    a. *Tai Xi* (Ki 3)

    b. *Shui Quan* (Ki 5)

    c. *Jiao Xin* (Ki 8)

    d. *Zhu Bin* (Ki 9)

Answer: _____

Source: C-193, D-348

186. Which acupoint on the kidney channel is especially effective in clearing vacuity heat causing genital itching?

    a. The wood point

    b. The fire point

    c. The river point

    d. The uniting point

Answer: _____

Source: C-191, D-338

187. Due to its location and supreme yin nature, which acupoint on the kidney channel rapidly treats replete head wind?

    a. *Yong Quan* (Ki 1)

    b. *Tai Xi* (Ki 3)

    c. *Zhao Hai* (Ki 6)

    d. *Ying Gu* (Ki 10)

Answer: _____

Source: C-191, D-336

188. Identify the alarm point of the kidney channel.

    a. *Shen Shu* (Bl 23)

    b. *Guan Yuan* (CV 4)

    c. *Tai Xi* (Ki 3)

    d. *Jing Men* (GB 25)

Answer: _____

Source: C-215, D-442

189. Which acupoint on the kidney channel is a master point of an extraordinary vessel?

    a. The earth point

    b. *Da Zhong* (Ki 4)

    c. The network point

    d. *Zhao Hai* (Ki 6)

Answer: _____

Source: C-193, D-344

190. What is the primary function of *Fu Liu* (Ki 7)?

    a. Treats heat in the head

    b. Treats irregular menstruation

    c. Treats edema

    d. Treats heel pain

Answer: _____

Source: C-193, D-346

191. Which acupoint, located close to the alarm point of the lung, unbinds the chest?

    a. *Ying Gu* (Ki 10)

    b. *Zhong Zhu* (Ki 15)

    c. *You Men* (Ki 20)

    d. *Shu Fu* (Ki 27)

Answer: _____

Source: C-198, D-362

192. Because it is the supplementation point on the kidney channel, which acupoint should be included to treat kidney yang vacuity and debility?

    a. *Ying Gu* (Ki 10)

    b. *Zhu Bin* (Ki 9)

    c. *Fu Liu* (Ki 7)

    d. *Yong Quan* (Ki 1)

Answer: _____

Source: C-193, D-346, F-123

193. Because of its ability to make the eyes close, which point on the kidney channel is used for all types of insomnia?

    a. *Rang Gu* (Ki 2)

    b. *Da Zhong* (Ki 4)

    c. *Zhao Hai* (Ki 6)

    d. *Jiao Xin* (Ki 8)

Answer: _____

Source: C-193, D-344

194. Identify the network point on the kidney channel.

    a. *Tai Xi* (Ki 3)

    b. *Da Zhong* (Ki 4)

    c. *Shui Quan* (Ki 5)

    d. *Fu Liu* (Ki 7)

Answer: _____

Source: C-192, D-342

195. Which of the following statements is *false* regarding *Tai Xi* (Ki 3)?

    a. It is the earth point.

    b. It treats lumbar pain.

    c. It is the draining point.

    d. It treats frequent and copious urination.

Answer: _____

Source: C-192, D-339

196. This point on the kidney channel secures the essence and thus is key for treating seminal emissions:

    a. *Da Zhong* (Ki 4)

    b. *Zhu Bin* (Ki 9)

    c. *Yin Gu* (Ki 10)

    d. *Da He* (Ki 12)

Answer: _____

Source: C-194, D-352

197. Like *Tian Shu* (St 25), *Huang Shu* (Ki 16), treats:

    a. Dysuria

    b. Constipation

    c. Irregular menstruation

    d. Replete cough

Answer: _____

Source: C-195, D-355

198. Which point on the kidney channel is best for treating impotence due to damp heat?

    a. The source point

    b. The spring point

    c. The fire point

    d. The horary point

Answer: _____

Source: C-194, D-350

Pericardium

199. Which of the following is the correct name for the pericardium channel?

    a. Hand *tai yang*

    b. Hand *shao yin*

    c. Hand *jue yin*

    d. Hand *tai yin*

Answer: _____

Source: C-199, D-367

200. Which acupoint on the pericardium channel is coupled with *Gong Sun* (Sp 4) to treat the penetrating vessel?

    a. The uniting point

    b. The source point

    c. The cleft point

    d. The network point

Answer: _____

Source: C-201, D-376

201. Identify the fire point on the pericardium channel.

    a. *Tian Chi* (Per 1)

    b. *Qu Ze* (Per 3)

    c. *Jian Shi* (Per 5)

    d. *Lao Gong* (Per 8)

Answer: _____

Source: C-201, D-380

202. Which of the following statements is *true* about *Zhong Chong* (Per 9)?

    a. It is the restraining point.

    b. It treats summerheat.

    c. It is the stream point.

    d. It treats vacuity pattern irregular menstruation.

Answer: _____

Source: C-202, D-382

203. Which acupoint on the pericardium channel is effective for treating blood patterns, especially acute blood stasis?

      a. *Tian Quan* (Per 2)

      b. *Qu Ze* (Per 3)

      c. *Xi Men* (Per 4)

      d. *Da Ling* (Per 7)

Answer: _____

Source: C-200, D-373

204. Because it is the water point, this acupoint on the pericardium channel is best known for its abilities for clearing heat from the qi, constructive, and blood aspects or divisions.

      a. The uniting point

      b. The stream point

      c. The source point

      d. The cleft point

Answer: _____

Source: C-200, D-372

205. What is the alarm point of the pericardium channel?

      a. *Jiu Wei* (CV 15)

      b. *Dan Zhong* (CV 17)

      c. *Da Ling* (Per 7)

      d. *Ge Shu* (Bl 17)

Answer: _____

Source: C-239, D-517

206. Which point on the pericardium channel is best for quelling nausea and vomiting resulting from a pattern of liver qi assailing the stomach?

      a. *Qu Ze* (Per 3)

      b. *Nei Guan* (Per 6)

      c. *Da Ling* (Per 7)

      d. *Zhong Chong* (Per 9)

Answer: _____

Source: C-201, D-376, F-11

207. Which point on the pericardium channel should be bled to treat windstroke?

      a. *Qu Ze* (Per 3)

      b. *Xi Men* (Per 4)

      c. *Nei Guan* (Per 6)

      d. *Zhong Chong* (Per 9)

Answer: _____

Source: C-202, D-382

208. Which point on the pericardium channel is best for treating insomnia resulting from heat ascending to harass the spirit?

      a. *Qu Ze* (Per 3)

      b. *Jian Shi* (Per 5)

      c. *Da Ling* (Per 7)

      d. *Zhong Chong* (Per 9)

Answer: _____

Source: C-201, D-378

Triple Burner

209. How many acupoints are on the triple burner channel?

    a. 19

    b. 23

    c. 25

    d. 27

Answer: _____

Source: C-208, D-412

210. Which acupoint is the intersection point of the triple burner and gallbladder channel and thus is the best for treating most diseases involving the ear?

    a. *Yang Chi* (TB 4)

    b. *Wai Guan* (TB 5)

    c. *Yi Feng* (TB 17)

    d. *Lu Xi* (TB 19)

Answer: _____

Source: C-207, D-408

211. Which acupoint on the triple burner channel is a heavenly window point?

    a. *Wai Guan* (TB 5)

    b. *Tian Jing* (TB 10)

    c. *Tian Liao* (TB 15)

    d. *Tian You* (TB 16)

Answer: _____

Source: C-206, D-407

212. Which acupoint on the triple burner channel is the master point of the yang linking vessel?

    a. *Ye Men* (TB 2)

    b. *Wai Guan* (TB 5)

    c. *Hui Zong* (TB 7)

    d. *Tian Jing* (TB 10)

Answer: _____

Source: C-396, D-203

213. Identify the source point on the triple burner channel.

    a. *Ye Men* (TB 2)

    b. The stream point

    c. The wood point

    d. *Yang Chi* (TB 4)

Answer: _____

Source: C-203, D-395

214. Which acupoint on the triple burner channel transforms phlegm and dissipates binding or nodules?

    a. The source point

    b. The well point

    c. The network point

    d. The uniting point

Answer: _____

Source: C-205, D-402

215. Which local acupoint on the triple burner channel is the most effective for treating pain and motor impairment of the shoulder and upper arm due to the contraction of external evils?

    a. *Yang Chi* (TB 4)

    b. *Wai Guan* (TB 5)

    c. *Jian Liao* (TB 14)

    d. *Yi Feng* (TB 17)

Answer: _____

Source: C-405, D-206

216. The point on the triple burner channel which is best for treating constipation of a replete nature is:

    a. *Wai Guan* (TB 5)

    b. *Zhi Gou* (TB 6)

    c. *Hui Zong* (TB 7)

    d. *San Yang Luo* (TB 8)

Answer: _____

Source: C-204, D-398

Sources: C=CAM, D=Deadman, F=Flaws, S=Shanghai

217. Which of the following statements is *false* regarding *Wai Guan* (TB 5)?

    a. It resolves wind heat contraction.

    b. It treats tinnitus.

    c. It is a key point in resolving *shao yang* headaches.

    d. It treats vacuity pattern diarrhea.

Answer: _____

Source: C-203, D-396

218. The restraining point on the triple burner channel is also the:

    a. Metal point

    b. Spring point

    c. Water point

    d. Uniting point

Answer: _____

Source: C-384, D-392

219. The stream point on the triple burner channel is a key distal point for the treatment of:

    a. Replete patterns of deafness

    b. Contraction of external heat evils

    c. Bursting pain in the eye

    d. Phlegm in the sinuses

Answer: _____

Source: C-203, D-393

220. Identify the alarm point of the triple burner channel.

    a. *Zhong Ji* (CV 3)

    b. *Shi Men* (CV 5)

    c. *San Jiao Shu* (Bl 22)

    d. *Wai Guan* (TB 5)

Answer: _____

Source: C-237, D-503

221. Which acupoint on the triple burner channel is indicated for treating facial paralysis, especially Bell's palsy?

        a. *Guan Chong* (TB 1)

        b. *Zhong Zhu* (TB 3)

        c. *Wai Guan* (TB 5)

        d. *Si Zhu Kong* (TB 23)

Answer: _____

Source: C-208, D-412

222. What is the lower uniting point of the triple burner channel?

        a. *Tian Jing* (TB 10)

        b. *Xia Ju Xu* (St 39)

        c. *Wei Yang* (Bl 39)

        d. *Wei Zhong* (Bl 40)

Answer: _____

Source: C-298, D-184

223. This acupoint on the triple burner channel is one of three in close proximity to the tragus which treat a wide variety of ear diseases:

        a. *Guan Chong* (TB 1)

        b. *Yi Feng* (TB 17)

        c. *Qi Mai* (TB 18)

        d. *Er Men* (TB 21)

Answer: _____

Source: C-208, D-410

Gallbladder

224. How many acupoints are on the gallbladder channel?

    a. 40

    b. 44

    c. 45

    d. 60

Answer: _____

Source: C-221, D-464

225. Which acupoint on the gallbladder channel located near the temple is a key one for managing migraine headaches?

    a. *Tong Zi Liao* (GB 1)

    b. *Ting Hui* (GB 2)

    c. *Shuai Gu* (GB 8)

    d. *Zu Ling Qi* (GB 41)

Answer: _____

Source: C-211, D-427

226. This acupoint on the gallbladder channel treats both *yang ming* and *shao yang* headaches affecting the eye:

    a. *Shuai Gu* (GB 8)

    b. *Yang Bai* (GB 14)

    c. *Feng Chi* (GB 20)

    d. *Jian Jing* (GB 21)

Answer: _____

Source: C-212, D-432

227. Which acupoint on the gallbladder channel is often paired with *Wai Guan* (TB 5) to treat the girdling vessel?

    a. The stream point

    b. The source point

    c. The network point

    d. The fire point

Answer: _____

Source: C-220, D-460

228. Originally used for rabies, this cleft point on the gallbladder channel continues to be effective in treating rage and manias:

    a. *Yang Ling Quan* (GB 34)

    b. *Yang Jiao* (GB 35)

    c. *Wai Qiu* (GB 36)

    d. *Guang Ming* (GB 37)

Answer: _____

Source: C-219, D-453

229. Which point on the gallbladder channel is effective in treating severe, generalized pruritus?

    a. The uniting point

    b. *Feng Shi* (GB 31)

    c. The network point

    d. *Yang Fu* (GB 38)

Answer: _____

Source: C-218, D-448

230. *Yang Jiao* (GB 35) is the cleft point of which extraordinary vessel?

    a. The girdling vessel

    b. The yang springing vessel

    c. The governing vessel

    d. The yang linking vessel

Answer: _____

Source: C-219, D-452

231. Identify the source point on the gallbladder channel.

    a. *Yang Ling Quan* (GB 34)

    b. *Guang Ming* (GB 37)

    c. *Qiu Xu* (GB 40)

    d. *Di Wu Hui* (GB 42)

Answer: _____

Source: C-220, D-458

232. Which local acupoint on the gallbladder channel, along with points on the triple burner and small intestine channels, treats a wide variety of diseases involving the ear?

    a. *Tong Zi Liao* (GB 1)

    b. *Ting Hui* (GB 2)

    c. *Zu Lin Qi* (GB 41)

    d. *Xia Xi* (GB 43)

Answer: _____

Source: C-209, D-422

233. Which acupoint on the gallbladder channel is effective for dispelling wind evils in the exterior?

    a. *Feng Chi* (GB 21)

    b. *Wai Qiu* (GB 36)

    c. *Qiu Xu* (GB 40)

    d. *Zu Lin Qi* (GB 41)

Answer: _____

Source: C-213, D-436

234. At which acupoint does the gallbladder channel intersect the girdling vessel?

    a. *Guang Ming* (GB 37)

    b. *Yang Ling Quan* (GB 34)

    c. *Huan Tiao* (GB 30)

    d. *Dai Mai* (GB 26)

Answer: _____

Source: C-216, D-443

235. Which acupoint on the gallbladder channel is the alarm point of the kidney channel?

    a. The network point

    b. The cleft point

    c. *Ri Yue* (GB 24)

    d. *Jing Men* (GB 25)

Answer: _____

Source: C-215, D-442

236. Which acupoint on the gallbladder channel is the primary point for treating hip pain of any etiology?

    a. *Zu Lin Qi* (GB 41)

    b. *Xuan Zhong* (GB 39)

    c. *Yang Ling Quan* (GB 34)

    d. *Huan Tiao* (GB 30)

Answer: _____

Source: C-217, D-446

237. Which of the following statements is *false* regarding *Yang Ling Quan* (GB 34)?

    a. It is the uniting point on the gallbladder channel.

    b. It is the master point of the sinews.

    c. It is used to treat a sweet taste in the mouth.

    d. It is the earth point.

Answer: _____

Source: C-218, D-450

238. Identify the alarm point of the gallbladder channel.

    a. *Ju Que* (CV 14)

    b. *Zhong Ting* (CV 16)

    c. *Ri Yue* (GB 24)

    d. *Jing Men* (GB 25)

Answer: _____

Source: C-215, D-441

239. Which acupoint on the gallbladder channel is contraindicated in the early trimesters of pregnancy?

    a. *Qiu Xu* (GB 40)

    b. *Guang Ming* (GB 37)

    c. *Yang Ling Quan* (GB 34)

    d. *Jian Jing* (GB 21)

Answer: _____

Source: C-214, D-438

240. Which acupoint on the gallbladder channel is the master point of marrow?

    a. *Dai Mai* (GB 26)

    b. *Ju Liao* (GB 29)

    c. *Xuan Zhong* (GB 39)

    d. *Xia Xi* (GB 43)

Answer: _____

Source: C-220, D-456

241. Which acupoint on the gallbladder channel brightens the eyes and treats eye itching and night blindness?

    a. The network point

    b. The cleft point

    c. The fire point

    d. The water point

Answer: _____

Source: C-219, D-454

242. Which acupoint on the gallbladder channel is most effective in treating both red and white vaginal discharge?

    a. *Yang Ling Quan* (GB 34)

    b. *Ju Liao* (GB 29)

    c. *Dai Mai* (GB 26)

    d. *Ri Yue* (GB 24)

Answer: _____

Source: C-216, D-443

243. For treating neck and shoulder pain involving the trapezius muscles, which acupoint on the gall-bladder channel is most effective?

> a. *Jian Jing* (GB 21)
>
> b. *Huan Tiao* (GB 30)
>
> c. *Yang Ling Quan* (GB 34)
>
> d. *Zu Lin Qi* (GB 41)

Answer: _____

Source: C-214, D-438

Liver

244. The primary use of xi guan (Liv 7) is to treat:

    a. Damp heat in the lower burner

    b. Knee pain

    c. Plumpit qi

    d. Menstrual disorders

Answer: _____

Source: C-223, D-484

245. Identify the alarm point of the liver channel.

    a. *Gan Shu* (Bl 18)

    b. *Shang Wan* (CV 13)

    c. *Zhang Men* (Liv 13)

    d. *Qi Men* (Liv 14)

Answer: _____

Source: C-226, D-490

246. Which acupoint on the liver channel is a master point?

    a. *Tai Chong* (Liv 3)

    b. *Li Gou* (Liv 5)

    c. *Zhang Men* (Liv 13)

    d. *Qi Men* (Liv 14)

Answer: _____

Source: C-226, D-488

247. Which acupoint on the liver channel is especially effective for treating genital itching?

    a. The source point

    b. The network point

    c. The wood point

    d. The uniting point

Answer: _____

Source: C-223, D-482

248. For a pattern of liver fire attacking the lungs, which point on the liver channel should be included in the prescription to clear the replete heat?

    a. *Xing Jian* (Liv 2)

    b. *Tai Chong* (Liv 3)

    c. *Zhong Du* (Liv 6)

    d. *Qu Quan* (Liv 8)

Answer: _____

Source: C-221, D-474, F-22

249. Which of the following is the correct name for the liver channel?

    a. Foot *tai yin*

    b. Hand *jue yin*

    c. Foot *jue yin*

    d. Hand *shao yin*

Answer: _____

Source: C-221, D-469

250. For a vacuity pattern involving both the liver blood and kidney yin, which acupoint should be selected to nourish the blood and yin?

    a. *Xing Jian* (Liv 2)

    b. *Tai Chong* (Liv 3)

    c. *Zhong Feng* (Liv 4)

    d. *Qu Quan* (Liv 8)

Answer: _____

Source: C-223, D-485, F-27

251. Which of the following is *false* regarding the earth point on the liver channel?

    a. It is the source point.

    b. It should not be used at any time during pregnancy.

    c. It is often paired with *He Gu* (LI 4) for treating replete patterns of headache.

    d. It treats a variety of urinary tract disorders.

Answer: _____

Source: C-222, D-477

252. For severe uterine bleeding, which point on the liver channel should be selected?

    a. *Da Dun* (Liv 1)

    b. *Tai Chong* (Liv 3)

    c. *Zhong Du* (Liv 6)

    d. *Zu Wu Li* (Liv 10)

Answer: _____

Source: C-221, D-473

253. The metal point on the liver channel is also the:

    a. Draining point

    b. Restraining point

    c. Supplementing point

    d. Horary point

Answer: _____

Source: C-222, D-481

254. For a pattern of depressive liver fire, what acupoint on the liver channel is often added to *Xing Jian* (Liv 2) with a through-and-through technique to resolve this condition?

    a. The uniting point

    b. The spring point

    c. The source point

    d. The metal point

Answer: _____

Source: C-222, D-477, F-21

255. Identify the horary point on the liver channel.

    a. *Da Dun* (Liv 1)

    b. *Xing Jian* (Liv 2)

    c. *Tai Chong* (Liv 3)

    d. *Qu Quan* (Liv 8)

Answer: _____

Source: C-384, D-473

256. Which point on the liver channel is the grandparent point?

     a. *Xing Jian* (Liv 2)

     b. *Tai Chong* (Liv 3)

     c. *Zhong Feng* (Liv 4)

     d. *Qu Quan* (Liv 8)

Answer: _____

Source: C-384, D-480

257. How many points are on the liver channel?

     a. 9

     b. 12

     c. 13

     d. 14

Answer: _____

Source: C-226, D-490

258. Which acupoint on the liver channel is the master point of the viscera?

     a. *Tai Chong* (Liv 3)

     b. *Li Gou* (Liv 5)

     c. *Zhang Men* (Liv 13)

     d. *Qi Men* (Liv 14)

Answer: _____

Source: C-226, D-488

Conception Vessel

259. How many alarm points are located on the conception vessel?

    a. 5

    b. 6

    c. 7

    d. Cannot be determined

Answer: _____

Source: C-393, D-43

260. *Tian Tu* (CV 22) is most commonly used for the treatment of:

    a. Menstrual disorders

    b. Plum pit qi

    c. Diarrhea

    d. Mental disorders, especially manias

Answer: _____

Source: C-240, D-522

261. The conception vessel contains two master points. One is the master point of the bowels; the other is:

    a. The master point of the blood

    b. *Guan Yuan* (CV 4)

    c. The master point of the sinews

    d. *Dan Zhong* (CV 17)

Answer: _____

Source: C-239, D-517

262. Which acupoint on the conception vessel is best for treating heart pain?

    a. *Qi Hai* (CV 6)

    b. *Shen Que* (CV 8)

    c. *Zhong Wan* (CV 12)

    d. *Ju Que* (CV 14)

Answer: _____

Source: C-239, D-514

263.   Which point on the conception vessel is the master point of the bowels?

    a. *Zhong Ji* (CV 3)

    b. *Guan Yuan* (CV 4)

    c. *Qi Hai* (CV 6)

    d. *Zhong Wan* (CV 12)

Answer: _____

Source: C-238, D-511

264.   Which of the following statements is *false* regarding *Qi Hai* (CV 6)?

    a. It supplements the original qi.

    b. It supplements the kidneys and invigorates yang.

    c. It is an intersection point of the conception vessel and spleen channel.

    d. It treats uterine bleeding.

Answer: _____

Source: C-397, D-504

265.   What is the primary function of *Shui Fen* (CV 9)?

    a. It treats constipation.

    b. It treats water swelling.

    c. It treats headache of any etiology.

    d. It treats replete cold patterns.

Answer: _____

Source: C-238, D-508

266.   Identify the stream point of the conception vessel.

    a. *Hui Yin* (CV 1)

    b. *Guan Yuan* (CV 4)

    c. *Shen Que* (CV 8)

    d. Extraordinary vessels do not have unique transport points.

Answer: _____

Source: C-384, D-29

267. Which of the following statements is *true* regarding *Shen Que* (CV 8)?

    a. It should be needled obliquely.

    b. Moxa on this point is forbidden.

    c. It is a primary point for rescuing yang desertion.

    d. It treats severe constipation involving repletion patterns.

Answer: _____

Source: C-238, D-508

268. In addition to treating pain and fullness in the chest, *Dan Zhong* (CV 17) treats:

    a. Insufficient lactation

    b. Sore throat

    c. Painful menses

    d. Groin pain

Answer: _____

Source: C-239, D-517

269. What is the primary function of *Qu Gu* (CV 2)?

    a. It treats rectal pain.

    b. It treats retention and dribbling of urine.

    c. It treats disorders of the large intestine.

    d. It treats calf pain.

Answer: _____

Source: C-235, D-498

270. Which of the following acupoints on the conception vessel would be best suited for treating vacuity conditions involving the female reproductive system?

    a. *Shang Wan* (CV 13)

    b. *Xia Wan* (CV 10)

    c. *Guan Yuan* (CV 4)

    d. *Zhong Ji* (CV 3)

Answer: _____

Source: C-237, D-501

271. *Cheng Jiang* (CV 24) treats:

    a. Facial wind

    b. Gum pain and swelling

    c. Deviation of the eyes and mouth

    d. All of the above

Answer: _____

Source: C-241, D-524

272. Identify the network point of the conception vessel.

    a. *Hui Yin* (CV 1)

    b. *Xia Wan* (CV 10)

    c. *Jiu Wei* (CV 15)

    d. The conception vessel has no network point.

Answer: _____

Source: C-239, D-515

Governing Vessel

273. Which point on the governing vessel is effective in treating acne rosacea or "drinker's nose?"

    a. *Bai Hui* (GV 20)

    b. *Shang Xing* (GV 23)

    c. *Su Liao* (GV 25)

    d. *Dui Duan* (GV 27)

Answer: _____

Source: C-234, D-558

274. Which of the following statements is *false* regarding *Da Zhui* (GV 14)?

    a. It treats malaria.

    b. It is the intersection point of the governing vessel and the three foot yang channels.

    c. It treats breast conditions, especially insufficient lactation.

    d. It treats stiffness of the neck and spine.

Answer: _____

Source: C-231, D-545

275. Which acupoint on the governing vessel is best for treating jaundice of any etiology?

    a. *Ming Men* (GV 4)

    b. *Zhi Yang* (GV 9)

    c. *Da Zhui* (GV 14)

    d. *Bai Hui* (GV 20)

Answer: _____

Source: C-230, D-540

276. Identify the network point on the governing vessel.

    a. *Chang Qiang* (GV 1)

    b. *Ming Men* (GV 4)

    c. *Xuan Shu* (GV 5)

    d. *Ya Men* (GV 15)

Answer: _____

Source: C-227, D-534

277. Which of the following statements is *false* concerning *Ming Men* (GV 4)?

    a. It treats stiffness of the lumbar spine.

    b. It is the back transport point of the kidneys.

    c. It treats rectal prolapse.

    d. It regulates the yang qi of the body.

Answer: _____

Source: C-228, D-536

278. Which acupoint on the governing vessel is indicated for treating welling abscesses?

    a. *Bai Hui* (GV 20)

    b. *Da Zhui* (GV 14)

    c. *Shen Zhu* (GV 12)

    d. *Ling Tai* (GV 10)

Answer: _____

Source: C-231, D-541

279. The governing vessel has two sea points. The upper one is *Bai Hui* (GV 20). Identify the lower one.

    a. *Feng Fu* (GV 16)

    b. *Da Zhui* (GV 14)

    c. *Ming Men* (GV 4)

    d. *Yao Shu* (GV 2)

Answer: _____

Source: D-48

280. How many acupoints are on the governing vessel?

    a. 20

    b. 25

    c. 26

    d. 28

Answer: _____

Source: C-235, D-561

281. Which acupoint on the governing vessel has the primary function of disinhibiting the nose?

    a. *Ren Zhong* (GV 26)

    b. *Shang Xing* (GV 23)

    c. *Qian Ding* (GV 21)

    d. *Bai Hui* (GV 20)

Answer: _____

Source: C-234, D-556

282. Which acupoint on the governing vessel is effective for treating swelling and pain of the gums and lips?

    a. *Yin Jiao* (GV 28)

    b. *Dui Duan* (GV 27)

    c. *Ren Zhong* (GV 26)

    d. *Bai Hui* (GV 20)

Answer: _____

Source: C-235, D-561

283. Which of the following statements is *false* regarding *Bai Hui* (GV 20)?

    a. It treats wind stroke.

    b. It treats rectal prolapse.

    c. It is the intersection point of all the channels.

    d. It treats most headache conditions.

Answer: _____

Source: C-233, D-552

284. There are two acupoints on the governing vessel renowned for restoring consciousness, especially when the patient is intoxicated. One is *Ren Zhong* (GV 26); what is the other?

    a. *Cheng Qiang* (GV 1)

    b. *Ming Men* (GV 4)

    c. *Su Liao* (GV 25)

    d. *Yin Jiao* (GV 28)

Answer: _____

Source: C-234, D-558

285. *Chang Qiang* (GV 1) is an important point for the treatment of:

    a. Dysuria

    b. Hemorrhoids

    c. Painful menses

    d. Low back pain

Answer: _____

Source: C-227, D-534

286. Identify the cleft point on the governing vessel.

    a. *Yao Yang Guan* (GV 3)

    b. *Zhong Zhu* (GV 7)

    c. *Ji Zhong* (GV 6)

    d. None of the above

Answer: _____

Source: C-390, D-38

287. What is the primary function of *Jin Suo* (GV 8)?

    a. It treats back spasms.

    b. It treats acid reflux due to stomach vacuity.

    c. It treats replete patterns of diarrhea.

    d. It treats irregular menstruation.

Answer: _____

Source: C-230, D-540

Non-channel Points

288. This group of four acupoints quiets the spirit, extinguishes wind, and treats dizziness:

    a. *Ba Feng* (M-LE-8)

    b. *Ba Xie* (M-UE-22)

    c. *Si Shen Cong* (M-HN-1)

    d. *Si Feng* (M-UE-9)

Answer: _____

Source: C-243, D-565

289. To aid in the diagnosis and treatment of appendicitis, this acupoint would be palpated and needled if tender:

    a. *Dan Nang Xue* (M-LE-23)

    b. *Lan Wei Xue* (M-LE-13)

    c. *Xi Yan* (MN-LE-16)

    d. *Bai Chong Wo* (M-LE-34)

Answer: _____

Source: C-252, D-583

290. Which pair of acupoints, located on either side of the spine, would be needled to treat acute asthma?

    a. *Yao Yan* (M-BW-24)

    b. *Hua Tuo Jia Ji* (M-BW-35)

    c. *Wei Guan Xia Shu* (M-BW-12)

    d. *Ding Chuan* (M-BW-1)

Answer: _____

Source: C-245, D-571

291. This non-channel acupoint is commonly needled through-and-through to *Shuai Gu* (GB 8) to treat headache:

    a. *Yu Yao* (M-HN-6)

    b. *Qiu Hou* (M-HN-8)

    c. *Yin Tang* (M-HN-3)

    d. *Tai Yang* (M-HN-9)

Answer: _____

Source: C-242, D-565

292. This acupoint, located just superior to the patella, treats knee pain and weakness:

    a. *He Ding* (M-LE-27)

    b. *Xi Yan* (M-LE-16)

    c. *Bai Chong Wo* (M-LE-34)

    d. *Da Nang Xue* (M-LE-23)

Answer: _____

Source: C-252, D-582

293. Which set of acupoints are bled to treat pain and swelling of the tongue?

    a. *Jia Cheng Jiang* (M-HN-18)

    b. *San Jiao Jiu* (M-CA-23)

    c. *Jin Jin Yu Ye* (M-HN-20)

    d. *Ba Feng* (M-LE-8)

Answer: _____

Source: C-244, D-570

294. This non-channel acupoint is appropriate for nasal obstruction.

    a. *Er Jian* (M-HN-10)

    b. *Bi Tong* (M-HN-14)

    c. *Tai Yang* (M-HN-9)

    d. *Bai Lao* (M-HN-30)

Answer: _____

Source: C-244, D-568

295. In addition to *Yin Tang* (M-HN-3), which non-channel acupoint should be employed to treat severe insomnia?

    a. *Si Shen Cong* (M-HN-1)

    b. *Yi Ming* (M-HN-13)

    c. *Tai Yang* (M-HN-9)

    d. *An Mian* (M-HN-54)

Answer: _____

Source: C-244, D-569

296. Which non-channel acupoint on the lower extremities treats severe itching and intestinal parasites?

    a. *He Ding* (M-LE-27)

    b. *Xi Yan* (MN-LE-16)

    c. *Bai Chong Wo* (M-LE-34)

    d. *Ba Feng* (M-LE-8)

Answer: _____

Source: C-252, D-582

297. These four hand acupoints are pricked and squeezed to produce a yellowish fluid when treating a variety of childhood nutritional disorders:

    a. *Shi Xuan* (M-UE-1)

    b. *Si Feng* (M-UE-9)

    c. *Ba Xie* (M-UE-22)

    d. *Yao Tong Xue* (N-UE-19)

Answer: _____

Source: C-249, D-577

298. Which non-channel acupoints on the abdomen are moxaed to treat prolapse of the uterus and irregular menstruation?

    a. *Zi Gong* (M-CA-18)

    b. *San Jiao Jiu* (M-CA-23)

    c. *Qi Zhong* (M-CA-10)

    d. *Yi Jing* (M-CA-14)

Answer: _____

Source: C-248, D-575

299. For stiff neck, this non-channel acupoint is often employed:

    a. *Yao Tong Xue* (N-UE-19)

    b. *Luo Zhen* (M-UE-24)

    c. *Ya Tong* (N-UE-1)

    d. *Zhong Kui* (M-UE-16)

Answer: _____

Source: C-250, D-579

300. Which non-channel acupoint is used for the diagnosis and treatment of damp heat in the gallbladder channel?

      a. *Lan Wei Xue* (M-LE-13)

      b. *Huan Zhong* (M-BW-34)

      c. *Er Bai* (M-UE-29)

      d. *Dan Nang Xue* (M-LE-23)

Answer: _____

Source: C-253, D-584

301. This facial acupoint is best for treating twitching and drooping of the eyelid:

      a. *Qi Hou* (M-HN-8)

      b. *Yin Tang* (M-HN-3)

      c. *Yu Yao* (M-HN-6)

      d. *Bi Tong* (M-HN-14)

Answer: _____

Source: C-243, D-566

302. This set of non-channel acupoints treats diseases in all regions of the body and regulates the five viscera and six bowels:

      a. *Shi Qi Zhu Xia* (M-BW-25)

      b. *Hua Tuo Jia Ji* (M-BW-35)

      c. *Ba Xie* (M-UE-22)

      d. *Ba Feng* (M-LE-8)

Answer: _____

Source: C-245, D-573

303. Which non-channel acupoint should be needled to dissipate phlegm nodules?

      a. *Bai Lao* (M-HN-30)

      b. *Er Jian* (M-HN-10)

      c. *Jia Cheng Jiang* (M-HN-18)

      d. *Ding Chuan* (M-BW-1)

Answer: _____

Source: C-246, D-569

304. This non-channel acupoint is a classic treatment for hemorrhoids and rectal prolapse:

    a. *Zi Gong* (M-CA-18)

    b. *San Jiao Qiu* (M-CA-23)

    c. *Ti Tuo* (N-CA-4)

    d. *Er Bai* (M-UE-29)

Answer: _____

Source: C-250, D-580

305. Which of these non-channel acupoints treats anterior shoulder pain?

    a. *Ba Feng* (M-LE-8)

    b. *Ba Xie* (M-UE-22)

    c. *Jian Qian* (M-UE-48)

    d. *Luo Zhen* (M-UE-24)

Answer: _____

Source: C-249, D-579

306. These ten points are pricked to bleed in emergencies to restore consciousness:

    a. *Hua Tuo Jia Ji* (M-BW-35)

    b. *Si Feng* (M-UE-9)

    c. *Shi Xuan* (M-UE-1)

    d. *Ba Xie* (M-UE-22)

Answer: _____

Source: C-249, D-577

307. Which non-channel acupoint treats diabetes?

    a. *Ding Chuan* (M-BW-1)

    b. *Wei Guan Xia Shu* (M-BW-12)

    c. *Yao Yan* (M-BW-24)

    d. *Shi Qi Zhu Xia* (M-BW-25)

Answer: _____

Source: C-246, D-571

Ear Acupuncture

308. Which ear acupoint regulates excitation and inhibition of the cerebral cortex and is often used for anesthesia?

      a. Heart

      b. Brain Stem

      c. Neurogate (*Shen Men*)

      d. Sympathetic

Answer: _____

Source: S-485

309. Which ear acupoint regulates excitation and inhibition of the respiratory center, and can also be used for itching?

      a. Upper Lung

      b. Lower Lung

      c. Sympathetic

      d. Stop Wheezing

Answer: _____

Source: S-484

310. For pain of the hip and sacroiliac joint as well as for atrophy of the gluteal muscles, which ear acupoint should be used?

      a. Lumbago

      b. Buttocks

      c. Hip Joint

      d. Lumbar Vertebrae

Answer: _____

Source: S-482

311. The Thirst ear acupoint is useful in treating diabetes and _____.

    a. Polyuria

    b. Hypertension

    c. Loss of appetite

    d. Depression

Answer: _____

Source: S-483

312. The ear apex is used as an acupoint which is bled to treat _____.

    a. Digestive problems

    b. Replete heat conditions

    c. Vacuity cold conditions

    d. Incontinence

Answer: _____

Source: S-479

313. For treating the symptoms of Meniere's disease, which ear acupoint should be used?

    a. Pituitary

    b. Headache

    c. Vertigo

    d. Nausea

Answer: _____

Source: S-484

314. Which of these ear acupoints regulates metabolism and treats gynecological and urogenital diseases?

    a. Subcortex

    b. Adrenal

    c. Pituitary

    d. Endocrine

Answer: _____

Source: S-484

Sources: C=CAM, D=Deadman, F=Flaws, S=Shanghai

315. Which of these conditions is *not* treated by the Brain Stem ear acupoint?

    a. Hemiplegia

    b. Insomnia

    c. Meningeal swelling

    d. Neck spasm

Answer: _____

Source: S-484

316. In addition to obstetrical and gynecological disease, the Uterus ear acupoint also treats:

    a. Diarrhea

    b. Constipation

    c. Male sexual dysfunction

    d. Obesity

Answer: _____

Source: S-485

317. Because it relaxes the smooth muscles, Sympathetic is also useful for treating:

    a. Gall and urethral stones

    b. Constipation

    c. Enuresis

    d. Tetany

Answer: _____

Source: S-481

Sources: C=CAM, D=Deadman, F=Flaws, S=Shanghai

Mixed Channels
Logic

For each of the next ten questions, you will be given a list of four acupoints. Three of these acupoints have something in common; the fourth does not. Identify the acupoint which *does not* belong.

318. a. *Tai Yuan* (Lu 9)

   b. *Chong Yang* (St 42)

   c. *Jin Men* (Bl 63)

   d. *Shen Men* (Ht 7)

Answer: _____

319. a. *Zhong Fu* (Lu 1)

   b. *Xuan Zhong* (GB 39)

   c. *Guan Yuan* (CV 4)

   d. *Zhang Men* (Liv 13)

Answer: _____

320. a. *He Gu* (LI 4)

   b. *Gong Sun* (Sp 4)

   c. *Hou Xi* (SI 3)

   d. *Nei Guan* (Per 6)

Answer: _____

321. a. *Jin Men* (Bl 63)

   b. *Xi Men* (Per 4)

   c. *Pian Li* (LI 6)

   d. *Jiao Xin* (Ki 8)

Answer: _____

322.   a. *Tai Yuan* (Lu 9)

        b. *Tai Chong* (Liv 3)

        c. *Zhong Wan* (CV 12)

        d. *Dan Zhong* (CV 17)

Answer: _____

323.   a. *Feng Long* (St 40)

        b. *Da Bao* (Sp 21)

        c. *Jiu Wei* (CV 15)

        d. *Da Ling* (Pc 7)

Answer: _____

324.   a. *San Jian* (LI 3)

        b. *Wan Gu* (SI 4)

        c. *Tai Bai* (Sp 3)

        d. *Zu Lin Qi* (GB 41)

Answer: _____

325.   a. *Chi Ze* (Lu 5)

        b. *Zu San Li* (St 36)

        c. *Fu Liu* (Ki 7)

        d. *Shang Ju Xu* (St 39)

Answer: _____

326.   a. *Tai Chong* (Liv 3)

        b. *Qu Chi* (LI 11)

        c. *Xiao Hai* (SI 8)

        d. *Kun Lun* (Bl 60)

Answer: _____

327.   a. *Da Ling* (Pc 7)

      b. *Hou Xi* (SI 3)

      c. *Li Dui* (St 45)

      d. *Shan Qiu* (Sp 5)

Answer: _____

Pairs

In traditional Chinese acupuncture, there are many famous acupoint pairs that are used together to treat a variety of disease patterns. In the next ten questions, identify these pairs and their use.

328. For the treatment of either insomnia or somnolence, which acupoint is paired with *Zhao Hai* (Ki 6) and either supplemented or drained?

     a. *Hou Xi* (SI 3)

     b. *Shen Men* (Ht 7)

     c. *Shen Mai* (Bl 62)

     d. *Zu San Li* (St 36)

Answer: _____

Source: C-190, D-320

329. For anterior shoulder pain, which acupoint is traditionally paired with *Jian Yu* (LI 15)?

     a. *He Gu* (LI 4)

     b. *Jian Liao* (TB 14)

     c. *Tiao Kou* (St 38)

     d. *Ju Gu* (LI 16)

Answer: _____

Source: C-206, D-405

330. For knee pain, two acupoints located on the eyes of the patella are employed. One is a non-channel point, the other is:

     a. *He Ding* (M-LE-27)

     b. *Liang Qiu* (St 34)

     c. *Du Bi* (St 35)

     d. *Zu San Li* (St 36)

Answer: _____

Source: C-154, D-157

331. Which acupoint pair is needled to treat insufficient lactation?

    a. *Ru Zhong* (St 17), *Ru Gen* (St 18)

    b. *Ru Gen* (St 18), *Liang Qiu* (St 34)

    c. *He Gu* (LI 4), *Zu San Li* (St 36)

    d. *Shao Ze* (SI 1), *Dan Zhong* (CV 17)

Answer: _____

Source: C-167, 239, D-231, 517

332. For most ear diseases involving tinnitus or deafness, three local acupoints are chosen. One of these points is *Ting Hui* (GB 2). Name the other two.

    a. *Shang Guan* (GB 3), *Xia Guan* (St 7)

    b. *Ting Gong* (SI 19), *Er Men* (TB 21)

    c. *Wang Gu* (GB 12), *Yi Feng* (TB 17)

    d. *Tian Chong* (GB 9), *Jiao Sun* (TB 20)

Answer: _____

Source: C-173, 208, D-247, 410

333. To control either profuse sweating or lack of sweating, what pair of acupoints is employed?

    a. *He Gu* (LI 4), *Tai Chong* (Liv 3)

    b. *Lie Que* (Lu 7), *Chi Ze* (Lu 5)

    c. *He Gu* (LI 4), *Fu Liu* (Ki 7)

    d. *Chi Ze* (Lu 5), *Yin Ling Quan* (Sp 9)

Answer: _____

Source: C-140, 193, D-103, 347

334. For skin diseases, especially those involving rashes due to a replete condition, a pair of yang channel uniting points is often used. Identify these acupoints.

    a. *Qu Chi* (LI 11), *Zu San Li* (St 36)

    b. *Xiao Hai* (SI 8), *Tian Jing* (TB 10)

    c. *Yang Ling Quan* (GB 34), *Wei Zhong* (Bl 40)

    d. *Qu Chi* (LI 11), *Wei Zhong* (Bl 40)

Answer: _____

Source: C-142, 184, D-113, 299

335. For hemorrhoids, which pair of acupoints on the same channel are most commonly used together?

    a. *Hui Yin* (CV 1), *Qu Gu* (CV 2)

    b. *Cheng Shan* (Bl 57), *Fei Yang* (Bl 58)

    c. *Chang Qiang* (GV 1), *Yao Yang Quan* (GV 3)

    d. *Yang Ling Quan* (GB 34), *Xuan Zhong* (GB 39)

Answer: _____

Source: C-188, D-315, 316

336. The most famous pair of acupoints in traditional Chinese acupuncture is the "four gates." This pair of acupoints is needled bilaterally to treat a wide variety of symptoms caused by liver depression qi stagnation. What is this famous pair?

    a. *Lie Que* (Lu 7), *He Gu* (LI 4)

    b. *Hou Xi* (SI 3), *Shen Mai* (Bl 62)

    c. *He Gu* (LI 4), *Tai Chong* (Liv 3)

    d. *Lie Que* (Lu 7), *Tai Chong* (Liv 3)

Answer: _____

Source: C-140, 222, D-103, 477

Simple Prescriptions

Chinese acupuncture is known for its ability to simply and elegantly treat a wide variety of disease, often with one or two points. In the next 34 questions, select the acupoint which is the *best* choice for treating the pattern or symptoms described.

337. Which of the following acupoints would best treat general pain and aching affecting the entire body?

    a. *He Gu* (LI 4)

    b. *Da Bao* (Sp 21)

    c. *Tai Chong* (Liv 3)

    d. *Yang Ling Quan* (GB 34)

Answer: _____

Source: C-163, D-204

338. Which of these command points would best treat stiffness in the nape of the neck?

    a. *Lie Que* (Lu 7)

    b. *He Gu* (LI 4)

    c. *Zu San Li* (St 36)

    d. *Wei Zhong* (Bl 40)

Answer: _____

Source: C-137, D-83

339. For clearing febrile conditions, especially due to a wind evil contraction, which of these extraordinary vessel master points would be the best choice?

    a. *Lie Que* (Lu 7)

    b. *Shen Mai* (Bl 62)

    c. *Nei Guan* (Ki 6)

    d. *Wai Guan* (TB 5)

Answer: _____

Source: C-203, D-396

340. Which of these acupoints effectively treats acid regurgitation as well as trigeminal neuralgia?

      a. *Zu San Li* (St 36)

      b. *Gong Sun* (Sp 4)

      c. *Nei Ting* (St 44)

      d. *Quan Liao* (SI 18)

Answer: _____

Source: C-156, D-171

341. For most eye problems, especially itching and redness, which local acupoint is most effective?

      a. *Guan Chong* (SI 1)

      b. *Tai Yang* (M-HN-9)

      c. *Zhan Zhu* (Bl 2)

      d. *Guan Ming* (GB 37)

Answer: _____

Source: C-174, D-257

342. Which of these master points treats both wilting and spasm of the limbs?

      a. *Ge Shu* (Bl 17)

      b. *Dan Zhong* (CV 17)

      c. *Da Zhu* (Bl 11)

      d. *Xuan Zhong* (GB 39)

Answer: _____

Source: C-220, D-456

343. Which of these upper uniting points treats tennis elbow and dissipates phlegm nodules?

      a. *Xiao Hai* (SI 8)

      b. *Tian Jing* (TB 10)

      c. *Qu Ze* (Pc 3)

      d. *Shao Hai* (Ht 3)

Answer: _____

Source: C-205, D-402

344. Which alarm point stops both vomiting and diarrhea?

    a. *Tian Shu* (St 25)

    b. *Qi Men* (Liv 14)

    c. *Ri Yue* (GB 24)

    d. *Zhong Wan* (CV 12)

Answer: _____

Source: C-238, D-511

345. Which of these fire points effectively treats constipation from any etiology?

    a. *Yang Xi* (LI 5)

    b. *Da Du* (Sp 2)

    c. *Zhi Gou* (TB 6)

    d. *Xing Jian* (Liv 2)

Answer: _____

Source: C-204, D-399

346. Which of these acupoints treats *pruritus vulvae* and nourishes blood and yin?

    a. *Qu Quan* (Liv 8)

    b. *Qu Chi* (LI 11)

    c. *San Yin Jiao* (Sp 6)

    d. *Wei Zhong* (Bl 40)

Answer: _____

Source: C-223, D-485

347. Which of these horary points treats impotence caused by damp heat?

    a. *Zu Tong Gu* (Bl 66)

    b. *Zu Lin Qi* (GB 41)

    c. *Tai Bai* (Sp 3)

    d. *Tai Xi* (Ki 10)

Answer: _____

Source: C-194, D-350

348. Which of these acupoints is best for treating any type of jaundice?

    a. The network point of the gallbladder channel

    b. The uniting point of the spleen channel

    c. The source point of the small intestine channel

    d. The cleft point of the liver channel

Answer: _____

Source: C-168, D-235

349. Which extraordinary vessel master point is always indicated for any kind of heart pain?

    a. *Gong Sun* (Sp 4)

    b. *Lie Que* (Lu 7)

    c. *Wai Guan* (TB 5)

    d. *Nei Guan* (Per 6)

Answer: _____

Source: C-201, D-376

350. Which of these distal acupoints is best for treating a frozen shoulder?

    a. *Yang Ling Quan* (GB 34)

    b. *Tiao Kou* (St 38)

    c. *Kun Lun* (Bl 60)

    d. *Yang Lao* (SI 6)

Answer: _____

Source: C-155, D-163

351. Which of these acupoints is best for malposition of the fetus?

    a. *He Gu* (LI 4)

    b. *Kun Lun* (Bl 60)

    c. *Zhi Yin* (Bl 67)

    d. *San Yin Jiao* (Sp 6)

Answer: _____

Source: C-191, D-325

352. For freeing the flow of lactation, which acupoint is always included in the prescription?

    a. *Shao Ze* (SI 1)

    b. *Tai Chong* (Liv 3)

    c. *Zu Lin Qi* (GB 41)

    d. *San Yin Jiao* (Sp 6)

Answer: _____

Source: C-161, D-231

353. Which acupoint is the empirical point for treating boils?

    a. *Qu Chi* (LI 11)

    b. *Xue Hai* (Sp 10)

    c. *Wei Zhong* (Bl 40)

    d. *Ling Tai* (GV 10)

Answer: _____

Source: C-230, D-541

354. Which cleft point treats both lumbar strain and cataracts?

    a. *Shui Quan* (Ki 5)

    b. *Jin Men* (Bl 63)

    c. *Yang Lao* (SI 6)

    d. *Wai Qiu* (GB 36)

Answer: _____

Source: C-168, D-237

355. Which of the following sea points treats blurred vision and dizziness?

    a. *Shang Ju Xu* (St 39)

    b. *Feng Fu* (GV 16)

    c. *Qi Chong* (St 30)

    d. *Dan Zhong* (CV 17)

Answer: _____

Source: C-233, D-548

Sources: C=CAM, D=Deadman, F=Flaws, S=Shanghai

356. For diarrhea, which of the following points would be moxaed but never needled?

    a. *Zu San Li* (St 36)

    b. *Tian Shu* (St 35)

    c. *San Jiao Jiu* (M-CA-23)

    d. *Zhong Wan* (CV 12)

Answer: _____
Source: D-575, S-376

357. Which of these acupoints relaxes the sinews and is forbidden during pregnancy?

    a. *Yang Ling Quan* (GB 34)

    b. *Kun Lun* (Bl 60)

    c. *San Yin Jiao* (Sp 6)

    d. *He Gu* (LI 4)

Answer: _____
Source: C-189, D-318

358. In addition to *Yin Bai* (Sp 1), which of these well points controls menorrhagia?

    a. *Da Dun* (Liv 1)

    b. *Yong Quan* (Ki 1)

    c. *Guan Chong* (TB 1)

    d. *Shao Ze* (SI 1)

Answer: _____
Source: C-221, D-473

359. Which extraordinary vessel master point is used to treat abdominal pain or distention due to qi stagnation, blood stasis, or damp obstruction?

    a. *Zu Lin Qi* (GB 41)

    b. *Gong Sun* (Sp 4)

    c. *Nei Guan* (Pc 6)

    d. *Zhao Hai* (Ki 6)

Answer: _____
Source: C-158, D-186

360. Which of these cleft points would be best for treating hemoptysis?

    a. *Di Ji* (Sp 8)

    b. *Jin Men* (Bl 63)

    c. *Kong Zui* (Lu 6)

    d. *Liang Qiu* (St 34)

Answer: _____

Source: C-137, D-82

361. One of these lower uniting points treats low back stiffness and pain. Identify it.

    a. *Zu San Li* (St 36)

    b. *Xia Ju Xu* (St 39)

    c. *Yang Ling Quan* (GB 34)

    d. *Wei Zhong* (Bl 40)

Answer: _____

Source: C-184, D-299

362. Which of these metal points treats edema and is also a supplementing point?

    a. *Xia Lian* (Lu 8)

    b. *Li Dui* (St 45)

    c. *Fu Liu* (Ki 7)

    d. *Ling Dao* (Ht 4)

Answer: _____

Source: C-193, D-346

363. Which of these command points controls sweating?

    a. *He Gu* (LI 4)

    b. *Wei Zhong* (Bl 40)

    c. *Zu San Li* (St 36)

    d. *Lie Que* (Lu 7)

Answer: _____

Source: C-140, D-103

364. In addition to *Fei Yang* (Bl 58), identify the network point which treats hemorrhoids.

  a. *Wai Guan* (TB 5)

  b. *Chang Qiang* (GV 1)

  c. *Da Zhong* (Ki 4)

  d. *Guang Ming* (GB 37)

Answer: _____

Source: C-227, D-534

365. Which acupoint on the upper back treats diabetes?

  a. *Da Zhu* (Bl 11)

  b. *Gao Huang* (Bl 43)

  c. *Wei Guan Xia Shu* (M-BW-12)

  d. *Ge Shu* (Bl 17)

Answer: _____

Source: C-246, D-571

366. Which of these acupoints best treats replete fire in the liver channel?

  a. *Bai Hui* (GV 20)

  b. *Qu Quan* (Liv 8)

  c. *He Gu* (LI 4)

  d. *Xing Jian* (Liv 2)

Answer: _____

Source: D-474, F-21

367. Which alarm point is generally incorporated in prescriptions for insufficient lactation?

  a. *Zhong Fu* (Lu 1)

  b. *Zhong Wan* (CV 12)

  c. *Ju Que* (CV 14)

  d. *Dan Zhong* (CV 17)

Answer: _____

Source: C-239, D-517

368. Which of these acupoints treats tidal fever and is the intersection point of at least three channels?

    a. *Hou Xi* (SI 3)

    b. *Wai Guan* (TB 5)

    c. *Da Zhui* (GV 14)

    d. *San Yin Jiao* (Sp 6)

Answer: _____

Source: C-231, D-545

369. Which of these acupoints is a heavenly window point which treats facial flushing?

    a. *He Gu* (LI 4)

    b. *Ren Ying* (St 9)

    c. *Fu Tu* (St 18)

    d. *Feng Fu* (GV 16)

Answer: _____

Source: C-147, D-137

370. Which of these earth points is a supplementation point that treats a racing heart?

    a. *Tai Yuan* (Lu 9)

    b. *Shen Men* (Ht 7)

    c. *Da Ling* (Pc 7)

    d. *Tai Xi* (Ki 3)

Answer: _____

Source: C-138, D-86

Point Location
Lung

371. The lung channel originates in the:

    a. Lung

    b. Upper burner

    c. Middle burner

    d. Lower burner

Answer: _____

Source: C-66, D-73

372. The lung channel connects with which other bowel or viscus?

    a. The small intestine

    b. The large intestine

    c. The heart

    c. The spleen

Answer: _____

Source: C-66, D-73

373. The network vessel of the lung channel emerges from which point?

    a. *Kong Zui* (Lu 6)

    b. *Lie Que* (Lu 7)

    c. *Jing Qu* (Lu 8)

    d. *Yu Ji* (Lu 10)

Answer: _____

Source: C-66, D-74

374. "Laterosuperior to the sternum at the level of the first intercostal space, 6 *cun* lateral to the midline." This describes the location of which acupoint?

      a. *Zhong Fu* (Lu 1)

      b. *Tian Fu* (Lu 3)

      c. *Chi Ze* (Lu 5)

      d. *Lie Que* (Lu 7)

Answer: _____

Source: C-135, D-76

375. Which is the correct description of the location of the cleft point of the lung channel?

      a. On the radial side of the thumb, about 0.1 *cun* posterior to the corner of the nail

      b. On the radial aspect of the midpoint of the first metacarpal bone, on the junction of the red and white skin

      c. On the palmar aspect of the forearm, on the line joining *Tai Yuan* (Lu 9), and *Chi Ze* (Lu 5), 7 *cun* above the transverse crease of the wrist

      d. On the medial aspect of the upper arm, 4 *cun* below the anterior of the axillary fold

Answer: _____

Source: C-137, D-82

376. Which of these acupoints is closest to the styloid process of the radius?

      a. *Chi Ze* (Lu 5)

      b. *Lie Que* (Lu 7)

      c. *Jing Qu* (Lu 8)

      d. *Tai Yuan* (Lu 9)

Answer: _____

Source: C-137, D-83

377. Which is the correct description of the location of the metal point of the lung channel?

      a. On the cubital crease of the elbow, in the depression at the radial side of the tendon of the *biceps brachii*

      b. One *cun* above the transverse crease of the wrist in the depression on the lateral side of the radial artery

      c. At the radial end of the transverse crease of the wrist, in the depression on the lateral side of the radial artery

      d. On the radial side of the thumb, about 0.1 *cun* posterior to the corner of the nail

Answer: _____

Source: C-138, D-86

378. Which of the following lung points is most distal to the elbow?

 a. *Xia Bai* (Lu 4)

 b. *Chi Ze* (Lu 5)

 c. *Kong Zui* (Lu 6)

 d. *Shao Shang* (Lu 11)

Answer: _____

Source: C-139, D-90

379. Which is the correct description of the location for *Tian Fu* (Lu 3)?

 a. On the lateral aspect of the arm, 3 *cun* below the end of the axillary fold, on the radial side of the *m. biceps brachii*

 b. On the medial aspect of the arm, 4 *cun* below the end of the axillary fold, on the radial side of the *m. biceps brachii*

 c. On the medial aspect of the arm, 4 *cun* below the end of the axillary fold, on the radial side of the *m. palmaris longus*

 d. On the medial aspect of the arm, 3 *cun* below the end of the axillary fold, on the radial side of the *m. biceps brachii*

Answer: _____

Source: C-136, D-78

380. "At the radial end of the transverse crease of the wrist in the depression on the lateral side of the radial artery." This describes the location of which acupoint on the lung channel?

 a. The spring point

 b. The source point

 c. The network point

 d. The alarm point

Answer: _____

Source: C-138, D-86

381. This acupoint is 5 *cun* below the cubital crease:

 a. *Chi Ze* (Lu 5)

 b. *Kong Zui* (Lu 6)

 c. *Lie Que* (Lu 7)

 d. *Jing Qu* (Lu 8)

Answer: _____

Source: C-136, D-80

382. Which of these acupoints is most proximal to the clavicle?

    a. *Zhong Fu* (Lu 1)

    b. *Yun Men* (Lu 2)

    c. *Shao Shang* (Lu 11)

    d. None of the above

Answer: _____

Source: C-136, D-77

383. What is the caution on needling *Zhong Fu* (Lu 1)?

    a. Moxibustion is forbidden.

    b. Deep, perpendicular needling may cause pneumothorax.

    c. Vigorous twisting of the needle may rupture the subclavian artery.

    d. Deep needling may puncture the brachial nerve.

Answer: _____

Source: C-135, D-78

384. Which of these points is 6 *cun* superior to *Chi Ze* (Lu 5)?

    a. *Jing Qu* (Lu 8)

    b. *Xia Bai* (Lu 4)

    c. *Tian Fu* (Lu 3)

    d. None of the above

Answer: _____

Source: C-136, D-78

385. The draining point on the lung channel is closest to the _____?

    a. Clavicle

    b. Elbow

    c. Wrist

    d. Thumb

Answer: _____

Source: C-138, D-86

For the following questions, refer to the diagram on the next page:

386. Which of the following acupoints is the uniting point of the lung channel?

    a. A

    b. B

    c. C

    d. D

Answer: _____

Source: C-136, D-80

387. Which of these acupoints is closest to the clavicle?

    a. E

    b. B

    c. A

    d. None of the above

Answer: _____

Source: C-135, D-76

388. Which acupoint is the master point of the vessels?

    a. E

    b. D

    c. C

    d. A

Answer: _____

Source: C-138, D-86

389. If acupoint C is the cleft point on the lung channel, how far is it from point B?

    a. 4 *cun*

    b. 5 *cun*

    c. 6 *cun*

    d. 7 *cun*

Answer: _____

Source: C-137, D-82

Lung

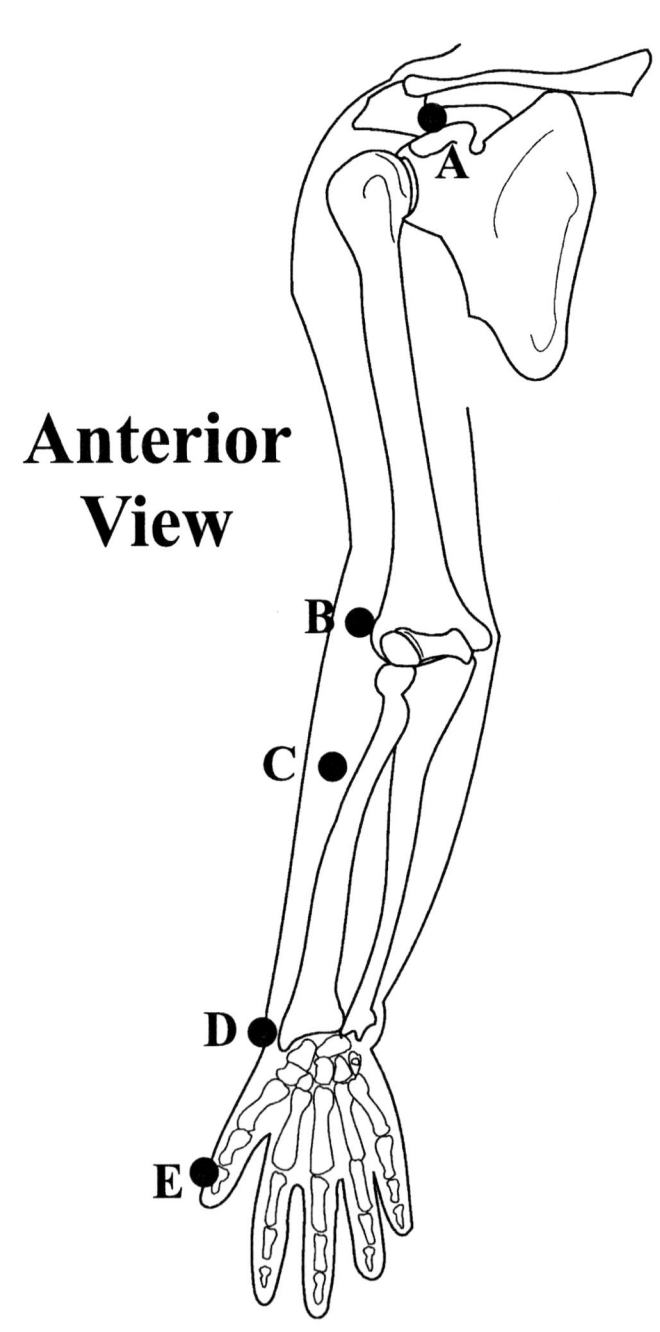

**Anterior
View**

390. Which of these acupoints is the wood point on the lung channel?

    a. B

    b. C

    c. D

    d. E

Answer: _____

Source: C-138, D-90

Large Intestine

391. The large intestine channel networks with what other viscus or bowel?

    a. Stomach

    b. Small Intestine

    c. Lung

    d. Heart

Answer: _____

Source: C-67, D-96

392. At which acupoint do the large intestine and stomach channels intersect?

    a. *Shang Yang* (LI 1)

    b. *He Gu* (LI 4)

    c. *Pian Li* (LI 6)

    d. *Ying Xiang* (LI 20)

Answer: _____

Source: C-68, D-96

393. "On the dorsum of the hand between the first and second metacarpal bones, approximately in the middle of the second metacarpal bone on the radial side." This describes the location of which acupoint on the large intestine channel?

    a. The spring point

    b. The source point

    c. The water point

    d. The cleft point

Answer: _____

Source: C-140, D-103

394. Which acupoint on the large intestine channel is located 10 *cun* above the wrist?

    a. *Wen Liu* (LI 7)

    b. *Xia Lian* (LI 8)

    c. *Shang Lian* (LI 9)

    d. *Shou San Li* (LI 10)

Answer: _____

Source: C-142, D-111

395. Which point location description fits the network point of the large intestine channel?

    a. 3 *cun* above the wrist

    b. 9 *cun* below the uniting point

    c. 2 *cun* below the cleft point

    d. All of the above

Answer: _____

Source: C-141, D-108

396. Which point on the large intestine channel is found in the depression appearing at the anterior border of the acromioclavicular joint when the arm is in full abduction?

    a. *Bi Nao* (LI 14)

    b. *Jian Yu* (LI 15)

    c. *Ju Gu* (LI 16)

    d. *Tian Ding* (LI 17)

Answer: _____

Source: C-143, D-116

397. How many *cun* units are there between the uniting and river points of the large intestine channel?

    a. 5

    b. 9

    c. 12

    d. 15

Answer: _____

Source: C-140, 142, D-106, 112

398. The stream point on the large intestine channel is found closest to what part of the upper extremity?

    a. The upper arm

    b. The lower forearm

    c. The wrist

    d. The forefinger

Answer: _____

Source: C-140, D-102

399. Which is the correct description of the location for *Wen Liu* (LI 7) ?

    a. With the elbow flexed and the radial side of the arm upward, the point is on the line connecting *He Gu* (LI 4) and *Qu Chi* (LI 11), 5 *cun* above the crease of the wrist.

    b. With the elbow flexed and the radial side of the arm upward, the point is on the line connecting *Yang Xi* (LI 5) and *Qu Chi* (LI 11), 5 *cun* above the crease of the wrist.

    c. With the elbow flexed and the ulnar side of the arm upward, the point is on the line connecting *Yang Xi* (LI 5) and *Qu Chi* (LI 11), 5 *cun* above the crease of the wrist.

    d. With the elbow flexed and the radial side of the arm upward, the point is on the line connecting *Yang Xi* (LI 5) and *Qu Chi* (LI 11), 7 *cun* above the crease of the wrist.

Answer: _____

Source: C-141, D-109

400. Which point on the large intestine channel is located in the nasolabial groove?

    a. *Fu Tu* (LI 18)

    b. *He Liao* (LI 19)

    c. *Ying Xiang* (LI 20)

    d. None of the above

Answer: _____

Source: C-144, D-120

401. What structure does the practitioner need to avoid when needling *Yang Xi* (LI 5)?

    a. The "snuff box" area

    b. The cephalic vein

    c. The radial artery

    d. The ulnar artery

Answer: _____

Source: C-140, D-106

402. Which acupoint on the large intestine channel is most distal to the shoulder?

    a. *Ju Gu* (LI 16)

    b. *Jian Yu* (LI 15)

    c. *He Gu* (LI 4)

    d. *Shang Yang* (LI 1)

Answer: _____

Source: C-139, D-100

403. Which acupoint on the large intestine channel is the most proximal?

    a. The well point

    b. The brook point

    c. The stream point

    d. The source point

Answer: _____

Source: C-136, D-103

404. On the large intestine channel, how many *cun* units are there between the cleft point and *Shang Lian* (LI 9)?

    a. 3

    b. 4

    c. 5

    d. 7

Answer: _____

Source: C-141, 142, D-109, 110

405. Which acupoint on the large intestine channel is located between the tendons of the *m. extensor pollicus longus* and *brevis*?

    a. *He Gu* (LI 4)

    b. *Yang Xi* (LI 5)

    c. *Pian Li* (LI 6)

    d. *Qu Chi* (LI 11)

Answer: _____

Source: C-140, D-106

For the following questions, refer to the diagram on the next page:

406. Acupoint A is located at which anatomical landmark:

    a. The tip of the humerus

    b. The transverse cubital crease

    c. The "anatomical snuffbox"

    d. The head of the second metacarpal bone

Answer: _____

Source: C-142, D-112

407. Acupoint B is the network point of the large intestine channel. If acupoint C is the fire point, how many *cun* units are there between points B and C?

    a. 1

    b. 2

    c. 3

    d. 4

Answer: _____

Source: C-141, D-108

408. Which of these acupoints is the source point on the large intestine channel?

    a. E

    b. D

    c. C

    d. A

Answer: _____

Source: C-140, D-103

409. Which of these acupoints is most distal to the olecranon?

    a. A

    b. B

    c. C

    d. D

Answer: _____

Source: C-140, D-103

Large Intestine

**Posterior
View**

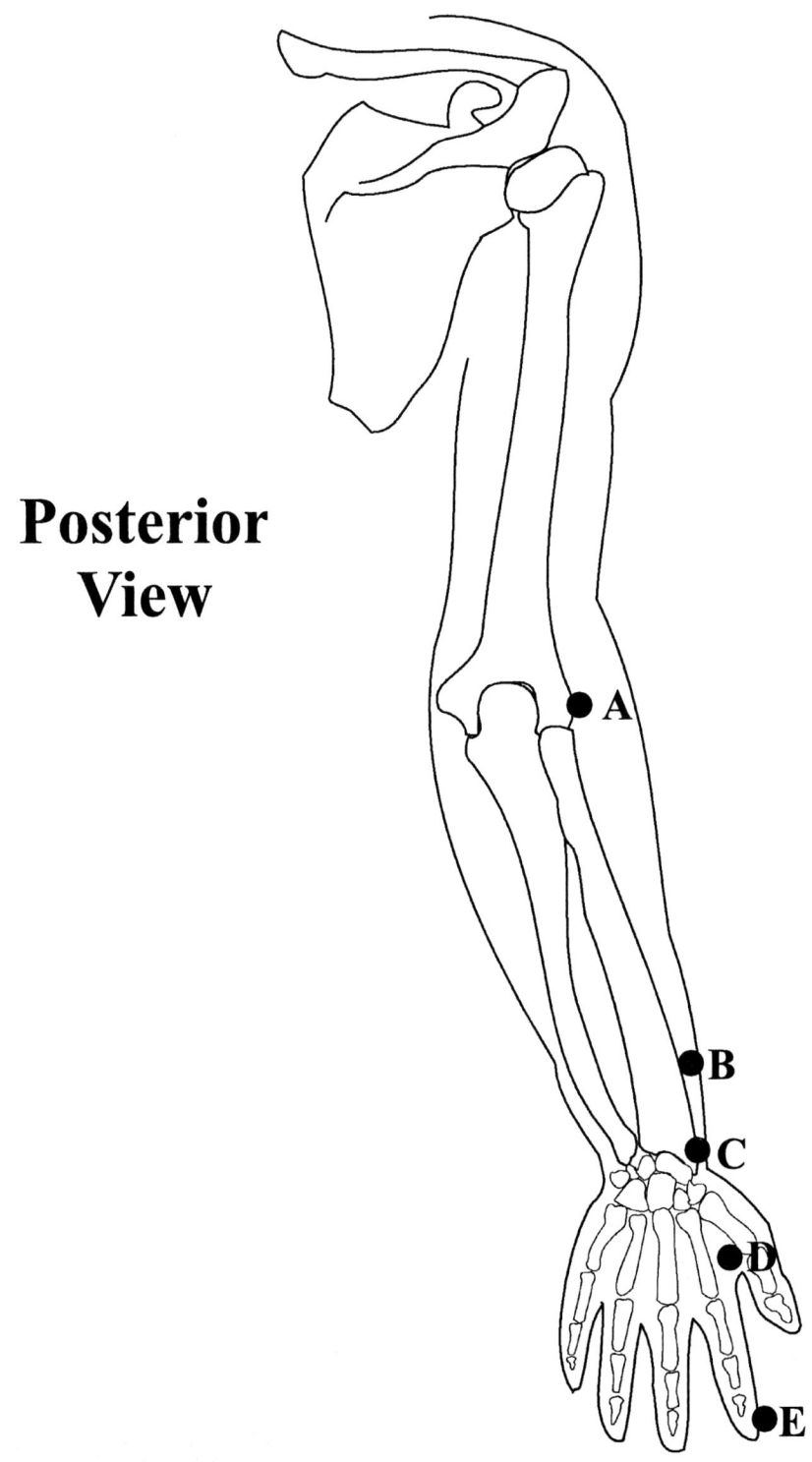

410. Acupoint C is the river point on the large intestine channel. How far is that point from the earth point on that channel?

     a. 16 *cun*

     b. 12 *cun*

     c. 4 *cun*

     d. 2 *cun*

Answer: _____

Source: C-142, D-112

Stomach

411. Where does the stomach channel begin?

    a. At the eye

    b. In the middle burner

    c. Between the second and third toes

    d. At the side of the nose

Answer: _____

Source: C-68, D-125

412. The stomach channel connects with what viscus or bowel?

    a. Spleen

    b. Heart

    c. Lung

    d. Large intestine

Answer: _____

Source: C-68, 69, D-126

413. What is the caution associated with needling *Cheng Qi* (St 1)?

    a. The eye must be looking straight ahead before needling.

    b. No manipulation of the needle should be attempted once it is inserted.

    c. To prevent injuring the eye, deep insertion into the socket is recommended.

    d. None of the above

Answer: _____

Source: C-145, D-130

414. What is the correct technique for needling *Tou Wei* (St 8)?

    a. Perpendicular, 0.5-1 *cun* depth

    b. Oblique, 0.5-1 *cun* depth

    c. Transverse, 0.5-1 *cun* depth

    d. Bleeding technique only

Answer: _____

Source: C-147, D-135

415. What is the distance between *Tiao Kou* (St 38) and the network point on the stomach channel?

    a. 1 *cun*

    b. 1.5 *cun*

    c. 1 finger width

    d. None, they are one and the same point

Answer: _____

Source: C-155, D-163, 165

416. How many *cun* units are there between the lower uniting points on the stomach and small intestine channels?

    a. 3

    b. 5

    c. 6

    d. 9

Answer: _____

Source: C-154, 155, D-158, 164

417. The alarm point of the large intestine is 2 *cun* lateral to what anatomical landmark?

    a. The umbilicus

    b. The upper edge of the pubic symphysis

    c. The point of the anterior superior iliac spine (ASIS)

    d. The lower border of the sternal notch

Answer: _____

Source: C-151, D-148

418. What is the caution associated with needling *Ren Ying* (St 9)?

    a. Avoid the jugular vein.

    b. Avoid the carotid artery.

    c. Avoid the *m. sternocleidomastoideus*.

    d. None of the above

Answer: _____

Source: C-147, D-137

419. Which acupoint on the stomach channel is lateral to the corner of the mouth, directly below the pupil of the eye?

     a. *Si Bai* (St 2)

     b. *Ju Liao* (St 3)

     c. *Di Cang* (St 4)

     d. *Da Ying* (St 5)

Answer: _____

Source: C-146, D-132

420. Which of these advisories does *not* apply to *Ru Zhong* (St 17)?

     a. No needling permitted

     b. No direct moxa to be applied

     c. Not to be used as a landmark

     d. All of the above

Answer: _____

Source: C-149, D-142

421. How many *cun* units are there between *Cheng Man* (St 20) and *Hua Rou Men* (St 24)?

     a. 2

     b. 3

     c. 4

     d. 5

Answer: _____

Source: C-150, 151, D-144, 147

422. The cleft point of the stomach channel is located 2 *cun* above what anatomical landmark?

     a. The pubic symphysis

     b. The 11th rib

     c. The anterior superior icheal spine (ASIS)

     d. The border of the patella

Answer: _____

Source: C-154, D-156

423. Which of these acupoints on the stomach channel is most distal?

    a. The source point

    b. The metal point

    c. The stream point

    d. The earth point

Answer: _____

Source: C-157, D-172

424. All of these acupoints involve needling into the *m. masseter* except:

    a. *Da Ying* (St 5)

    b. *Jia Che* (St 6)

    c. *Xia Guan* (St 7)

    d. All of the above are needled into the *m. masseter*

Answer: _____

Source: C-146, D-133-134

425. Which is the correct description of the location for *Zu San Li* (St 36)?

    a. 4 *cun* below *Du Bi* (St 35), 1 finger width from the anterior border of the tibia

    b. 3 *cun* below *Du Bi* (St 35), 2 finger widths from the anterior border of the tibia

    c. 3 *cun* below *Du Bi* (St 35), 1 finger width from the anterior border of the tibia

    d. 4 *cun* below *Du Bi* (St 35), 2 finger widths from the anterior border of the tibia

Answer: _____

Source: C-141, D-109

For the following questions, refer to the diagram on the next page:

426. On which of these acupoints is moxa forbidden?

    a. A

    b. B

    c. C

    d. E

Answer: _____

Source: C-149, D-142

427. Acupoint D is the lower uniting point of the large intestine channel. How far is it from the uniting point of the stomach channel?

    a. 3 *cun*

    b. 4 *cun*

    c. 8 *cun*

    d. 13 *cun*

Answer: _____

Source: C-154, D-162

428. Which of these acupoints is the alarm point of the large intestine?

    a. A

    b. B

    c. C

    d. E

Answer: _____

Source: C-151, D-148

429. Which of these acupoints is the fire point on the stomach channel?

    a. C

    b. D

    c. E

    d. None of the above

Answer: _____

Source: C-155, D-167

Stomach

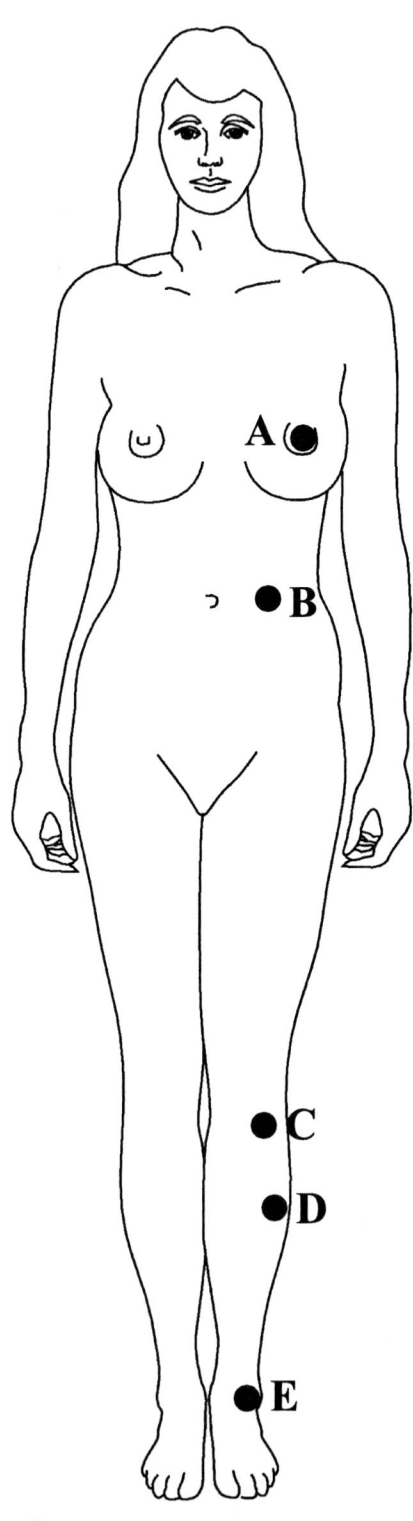

430. If acupoint C is the earth point on the stomach channel, how far is it from acupoint E?

     a. 8 *cun*

     b. 12 *cun*

     c. 13 *cun*

     d. 16 *cun*

Answer: _____

Source: C-154, D-158

Spleen

431. Where does the spleen channel begin?

    a. At the spleen

    b. Beside the stomach

    c. At the medial tip of the big toe

    d. At the lateral tip of the big toe

Answer: _____

Source: C-69, D-177

432. In addition to the stomach, the spleen channel networks with which viscus or bowel?

    a. Lung

    b. Large intestine

    c. Heart

    d. Small intestine

Answer: _____

Source: C-69, D-178

433. Which is the correct description for locating *Tai Bai* (Sp 3)?

    a. On the lateral side of the foot, proximal and inferior to the head of the first metatarsal bone

    b. On the medial side of the foot, proximal and inferior to the head of the first metatarsal bone

    c. On the medial side of the foot, in the depression distal and inferior to the base of the first metatarsal bone

    d. On the medial side of the ankle, in the depression midway between the tuberosity of the navicular bone and the tip of the medial malleolus

Answer: _____

Source: C-157, D-184

434. "4 *cun* lateral to the center of the umbilicus, lateral to the *m. rectus abdominis.*" This describes the location of which acupoint on the spleen channel?

      a. *Fu She* (Sp 13)

      b. *Fu Jie* (Sp 14)

      c. *Da Heng* (Sp 15)

      d. *Fu Ai* (Sp 16)

Answer: _____

Source: C-161, D-184

435. Which acupoint on the spleen channel is located in the fourth intercostal space?

      a. *Shi Dou* (Sp 17)

      b. *Tian Xi* (Sp 18)

      c. *Xiong Xiang* (Sp 19)

      d. *Zhou Rong* (Sp 20)

Answer: _____

Source: C-162, D-202

436. Which of these acupoints is *not* 4 *cun* lateral to the midline?

      a. *Fu Jie* (Sp 14)

      b. *Da Heng* (Sp 15)

      c. *Fu Ai* (Sp 16)

      d. *Shi Dou* (Sp 17)

Answer: _____

Source: C-161, D-201

437. How many *cun* units are there between *Yin Ling Quan* (Sp 9) and *Lou Gu* (Sp 7)?

      a. 4

      b. 6

      c. 7

      d. 8

Answer: _____

Source: C-159, D-192

438. What acupoint on the spleen channel is 10 *cun* below *Yin Ling Quan* (Sp 9)?

    a. *Shang Qiu* (Sp 5)

    b. *San Yin Jiao* (Sp 6)

    c. *Lou Gu* (Sp 7)

    d. *Di Ji* (Sp 8)

Answer: _____

Source: C-159, D-189

439. Which three channels intersect at *San Yin Jiao* (Sp 6)?

    a. Lung, heart, spleen

    b. Liver, gallbladder, spleen

    c. Liver, kidney, spleen

    d. Stomach, gallbladder, bladder

Answer: _____

Source: C-69, D-189

440. Which of these acupoints does *not* fall on the line which connects the spleen uniting point and the medial malleolus?

    a. *Yin Ling Quan* (Sp 9)

    b. *Di Ji* (Sp 8)

    c. *Lou Gu* (Sp 7)

    d. All of these acupoints fall on the line

Answer: _____

Source: C-159, D-193

441. Which acupoint is often located by resting the heel of the hand below the patient's patella and extending the thumb?

    a. *Xue Hai* (Sp 10)

    b. *Ji Men* (Sp 11)

    c. *Chong Men* (Sp 12)

    d. *Fu She* (Sp 13)

Answer: _____

Source: C-160, D-196

442. What anatomical structure runs beneath both *Ji Men* (Sp 11) and *Chong Men* (Sp 12) and requires caution on the part of the acupuncturist when needling these acupoints?

    a. The femoral nerve

    b. The inguinal vein

    c. The femoral artery

    d. The ilioinguinal nerve

Answer: _____

Source: C-160-161, D-197-198

443. What is the caution associated with needling *Da Bao* (Sp 21)?

    a. Deep, perpendicular insertion may puncture the intercostal artery.

    b. Shallow, transverse-oblique insertion may puncture the intercostal artery.

    c. Deep, perpendicular insertion may cause pneumothorax in thin patients.

    d. Shallow, transverse-oblique insertion may cause pneumothorax in thin patients.

Answer: _____

Source: C-163, D-204

444. Which of these acupoints is most proximal to the well point on the spleen channel?

    a. *Yang Ling Quan* (Sp 9)

    b. *San Yin Jiao* (Sp 6)

    c. *Shang Qiu* (Sp 5)

    d. *Gong Sun* (Sp 4)

Answer: _____

Source: C-160, D-194

445. The great network channel separates from the spleen channel at which acupoint?

    a. *Gong Sun* (Sp 4)

    b. *San Yin Jiao* (Sp 6)

    c. *Xue Hai* (Sp 10)

    d. *Da Bao* (Sp 21)

Answer: _____

Source: C-163, D-204

For the following questions, refer to the diagram on the next page:

446. Which of the acupoints pictured is the source point on the spleen channel?

    a. E

    b. D

    c. C

    d. B

Answer: _____

Source: C-157, D-184

447. Acupoint B is how many *cun* units lateral to the navel?

    a. 3

    b. 4

    c. 5

    d. 6

Answer: _____

Source: C-161, D-200

448. If acupoint C is the uniting point and acupoint D is the cleft point on the spleen channel, how many *cun* units are there between the two of them?

    a. 2

    b. 3

    c. 4

    d. 6

Answer: _____

Source: C-159, D-193

449. Acupoint A is *Shi Dou* (Sp 17). In what intercostal space is this acupoint located?

    a. 3rd

    b. 4th

    c. 5th

    d. 6th

Answer: _____

Source: C-161, D-201

Spleen

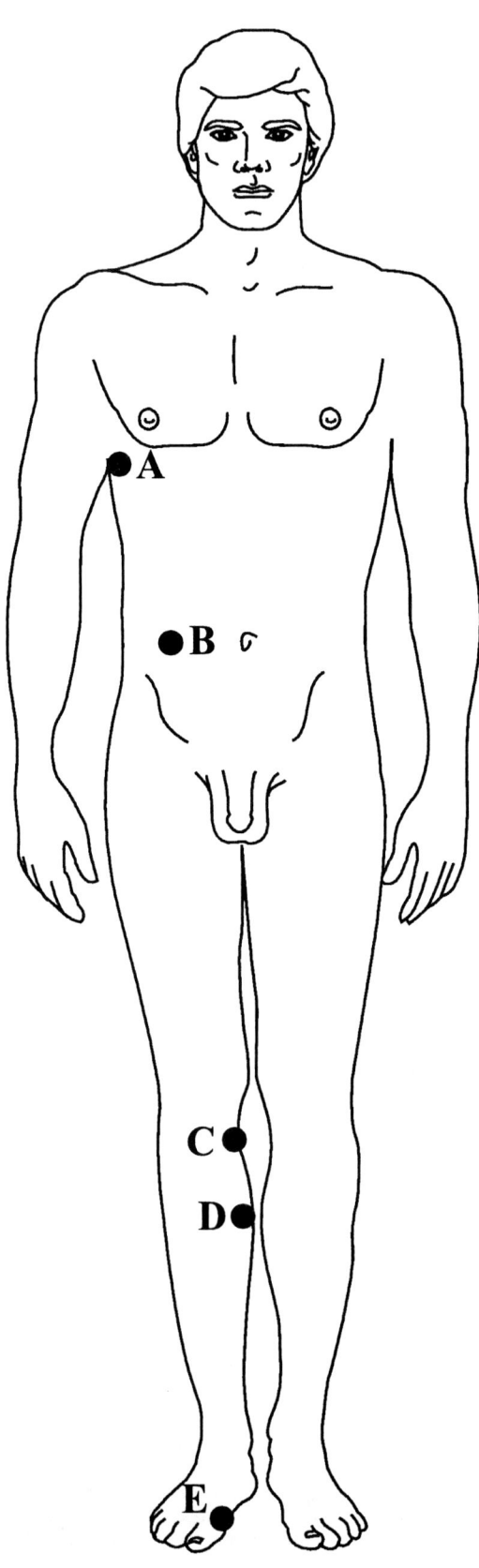

450. Which of the acupoints pictured is the most distal from the knee?

    a. B

    b. C

    c. D

    d. E

Answer: _____

Source: C-157, D-184

Heart

451. Where does the heart channel originate?

    a. In the heart

    b. Next to the left nipple

    c. In the pericardium

    d. At the little finger

Answer: _____

Source: C-69, D-209

452. "When the palm faces upward, the point is on the radial side of the *m. flexor carpi ulnaris*, 1 *cun* above the transverse crease of the wrist." This describes the location of which acupoint on the heart channel?

    a. *Ling Dao* (Ht 4)

    b. *Tong Li* (Ht 5)

    c. *Yin Xi* (Ht 6)

    d. *Shen Men* (Ht 7)

Answer: _____

Source: C-165, D-216

453. Which acupoint on the heart channel is 0.5 *cun* distal to *Tong Li* (Ht 5)?

    a. *Shao Hai* (Ht 3)

    b. *Ling Dao* (Ht 4)

    c. *Yin Xi* (Ht 6)

    d. *Shen Men* (Ht 7)

Answer: _____

Source: C-165, D-217

454. The uniting point of the heart channel is located near which anatomical structure?

    a. The little finger

    b. The thumb

    c. In the middle of the forearm

    d. The elbow

Answer: _____

Source: C-164, D-214

455. How many *cun* units are there between the source point and the river point of the heart channel?

   a. 0.5

   b. 1

   c. 1.5

   d. 2

Answer: _____

Source: C-165, D-215

456. Which is the proper technique for locating *Shao Fu* (Ht 8)?

   a. On the palm, in the depression between the 3rd and 4th metacarpal bones, where the tip of the little finger rests when a fist is made

   b. On the palm, in the depression between the 4th and 5th metacarpal bones, where the tip of the little finger rests when a fist is made

   c. On the palm, in the depression between the 4th and 5th metacarpal bones, where the tip of the 4th finger rests when a fist is made

   d. At the ulnar end of the transverse crease of the wrist in the depression on the radial side of the tendon of the *m. flexor carpi ulnaris*

Answer: _____

Source: C-166, D-221

457. Which of the following points on the heart channel is closest to the elbow?

   a. *Shen Men* (Ht 7)

   b. *Yin Xi* (Ht 6)

   c. *Tong Li* (Ht 5)

   d. *Ling Dao* (Ht 4)

Answer: _____

Source: C-165, D-215

458. What is the caution associated with needling *Shen Men* (Ht 7)?

   a. Take care not to puncture the radial artery.

   b. Needling too deeply will cause the premature obtaining of the qi.

   c. Avoid puncturing the ulnar artery.

   d. No moxa is permitted on this point.

Answer: _____

Source: C-166, D-219

459. The well point on the heart channel is located:

    a. On the ulnar side of the little finger

    b. On the radial side of the little finger

    c. On the inside of the elbow

    d. None of the above

Answer: _____

Source: C-166, D-222

460. Which of the following is the correct description for the location of *Ji Quan* (Ht 1)?

    a. When the elbow is flexed, the point is 3 *cun* above the medial end of the transverse cubital crease.

    b. With the elbow flexed, locate the point at the midpoint of the line connecting the medial end of the cubital crease and the medial epicondyle of the humerus.

    c. 1 *cun* lateral to the nipple in the 4th intercostal space

    d. When the upper arm is abducted, the point is in the center of the axilla on the medial side of the axillary artery.

Answer: _____

Source: C-164, D-212

For the following questions, refer to the diagram on the next page:

461. Which of these acupoints is the water point on the heart channel?

    a. A

    b. B

    c. D

    d. E

Answer: _____

Source: C-164, D-214

462. Which of these acupoints is the mother point on the heart channel?

    a. E

    b. D

    c. C

    d. B

Answer: _____

Source: C-166, D-221

463. Acupoint D is the draining point on the heart channel. Acupoint C is the metal point. How many *cun* units are there between the two acupoints?

    a. 0.5

    b. 1

    c. 1.5

    d. 2

Answer: _____

Source: C-165, D-215

464. Acupoint A is *Qing Ling* (Ht 2). If acupoint B is the uniting point on the heart channel, how many *cun* units separate acupoints A and B?

    a. 9

    b. 5

    c. 4

    d. 3

Answer: _____

Source: C-164, D-213

Heart

Anterior View

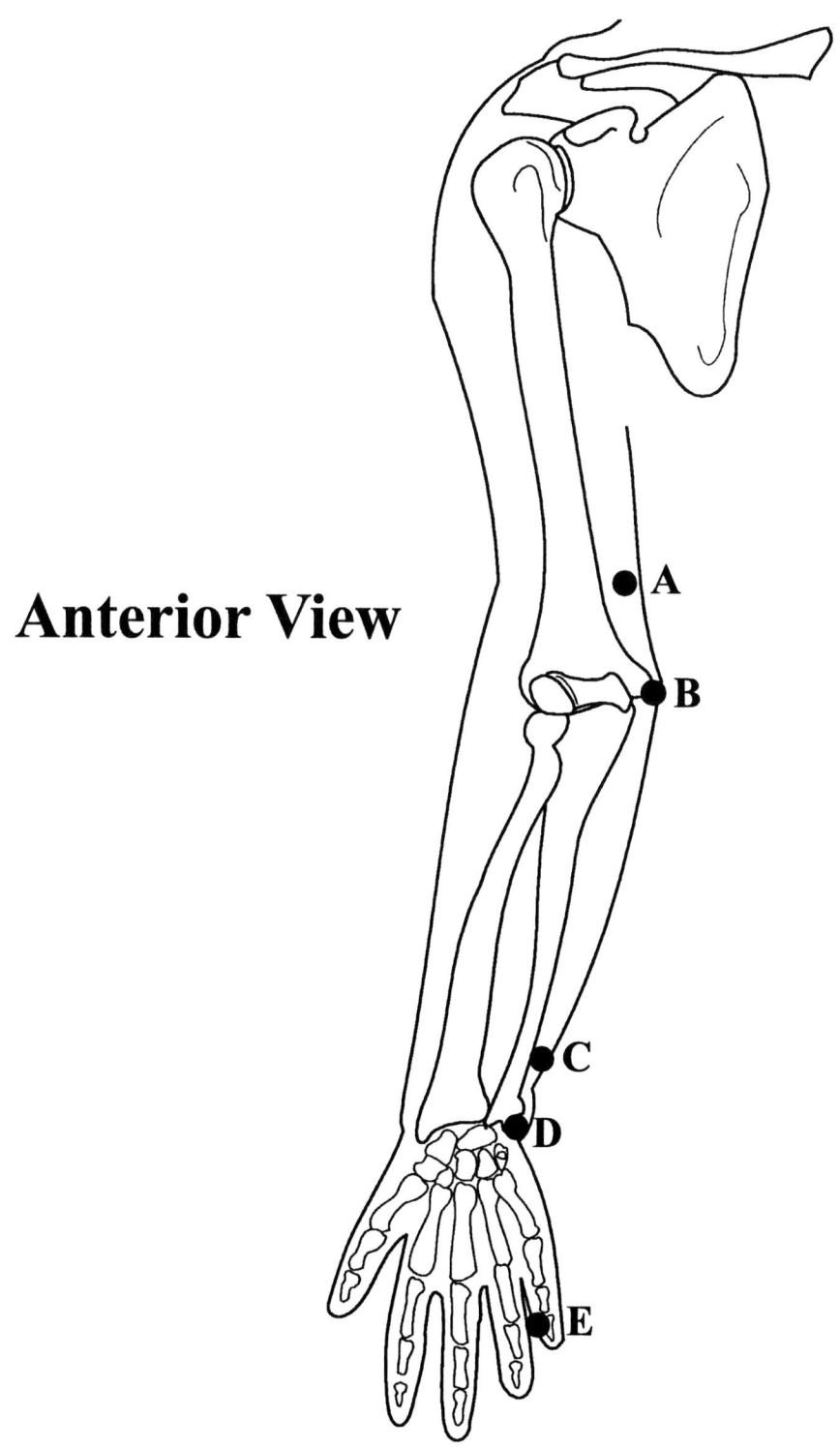

465. If acupoint B is the uniting point of the heart channel and acupoint D is the earth point, how many *cun* units are there between acupoints B and D?

    a. 8

    b. 9

    c. 10

    d. 12

Answer: _____

Source: C-120, D-63

Small Intestine

466. "When a loose fist is made, the point is on the ulnar end of the distal palmar crease, proximal to the 5th metacarpalphalangeal joint at the end of the transverse crease and the junction of the red and white skin." This describes the location of which acupoint on the small intestine channel?

    a. *Shao Ze* (SI 1)

    b. *Qiang Gu* (SI 2)

    c. *Hou Xi* (SI 3)

    d. *Wang Gu* (SI 4)

Answer: _____

Source: C-167, D-233

467. At which acupoint does the small intestine network channel separate from its primary channel?

    a. *Hou Xi* (SI 3)

    b. *Wang Gu* (SI 4)

    c. *Yang Lao* (SI 6)

    d. *Zhi Zheng* (SI 7)

Answer: _____

Source: C-168, D-169

468. How many *cun* units separate *Zhi Zheng* (SI 7) and *Xiao Hai* (SI 8)?

    a. 12 *cun*

    b. 8 *cun*

    c. 7 *cun*

    d. 5 *cun*

Answer: _____

Source: C-169, D-238

469. *Yang Lao* (SI 6) is found near what prominent anatomical structure?

    a. The second knuckle on the index finger

    b. The bony cleft on the radial side of the ulna

    c. The bony cleft on the ulnar side of the radius

    d. At the transverse crease of the wrist

Answer: _____

Source: C-168, D-237

470. Which of the following is the correct description for the location of *Tian Zong* (SI 11)?

    a. Directly above the posterior end of the axillary fold, in the depression inferior to the scapular spine

    b. On the scapula, in the depression of the center of the subscapular fossa, at the level of the 4th thoracic vertebra

    c. On the medial extremity of the suprascapular fossa, about midway between *Nao Shu* (SI 10) and the spinous process of the 2nd thoracic vertebra

    d. 3 *cun* lateral to the lower border of the first thoracic vertebra where *Tao Dao* (GV 13) is located

Answer: _____

Source: C-171, D-241

471. Which acupoint on the small intestine channel lies directly below the outer canthus, in the depression on the lower border of the zygomatic bone?

    a. *Tian Chuang* (SI 16)

    b. *Tian Rong* (SI 17)

    c. *Quan Liao* (SI 18)

    d. *Ting Gong* (SI 19)

Answer: _____

Source: C-173, D-246

472. How many *cun* units lie between the river point and the uniting point on the small intestine channel?

    a. 5

    b. 7

    c. 9

    d. 12

Answer: _____

Source: C-168, D-238

473. Which acupoint on the small intestine channel lies between the base of the fifth metacarpal bone and the triquetral bone?

    a. The water point

    b. The stream point

    c. The source point

    d. The cleft point

Answer: _____

Source: C-168, D-235

474. Which of these acupoints lies most proximal to *Xiao Hai* (SI 8)?

      a. *Shao Ze* (SI 1)

      b. *Zhi Zheng* (SI 7)

      c. *Jian Zhen* (SI 9)

      d. *Tian Zong* (SI 11)

Answer: _____

Source: C-169, D-240

475. Which one of the acupoints on the small intestine channel lies at the level of *Da Zhui* (GV 14)?

      a. *Tian Chuang* (SI 16)

      b. *Jian Zhong Shu* (SI 15)

      c. *Jian Wai Shu* (SI 14)

      d. *Qu Yuan* (SI 13)

Answer: _____

Source: C-172, D-244

For the following questions, refer to the diagram on the next page:

476. Acupoint A is in the center of the supraclavicular fossa and is the intersection point of the three yang hand channels. Which acupoint is it?

    a. *Tian Zong* (SI 11)

    b. *Bi Feng* (SI 12)

    c. *Qu Yuan* (SI 13)

    d. *Jian Wai Shu* (SI 14)

Answer: _____

Source: C-171, D-242

477. Acupoint C is the network point and lies *5 cun* proximal to acupoint D. Identify acupoint D.

    a. The spring point

    b. The wood point

    c. The source point

    d. The fire point

Answer: _____

Source: C-168, D-236

478. Acupoint B is located 1 *cun* above the posterior end of the axillary fold when the arm is adducted. Identify acupoint B.

    a. *Jian Zhen* (SI 9)

    b. *Nao Shu* (SI 10)

    c. *Tian Zong* (SI 11)

    d. *Bing Feng* (SI 12)

Answer: _____

Source: C-169, D-240

479. Acupoint E is located on the ulnar side of the little finger, about 0.1 *cun* from the corner of the nail. This makes it the:

    a. Stream point

    b. Water point

    c. Wood point

    d. Metal point

Answer: _____

Source: C-167, D-231

Small Intestine

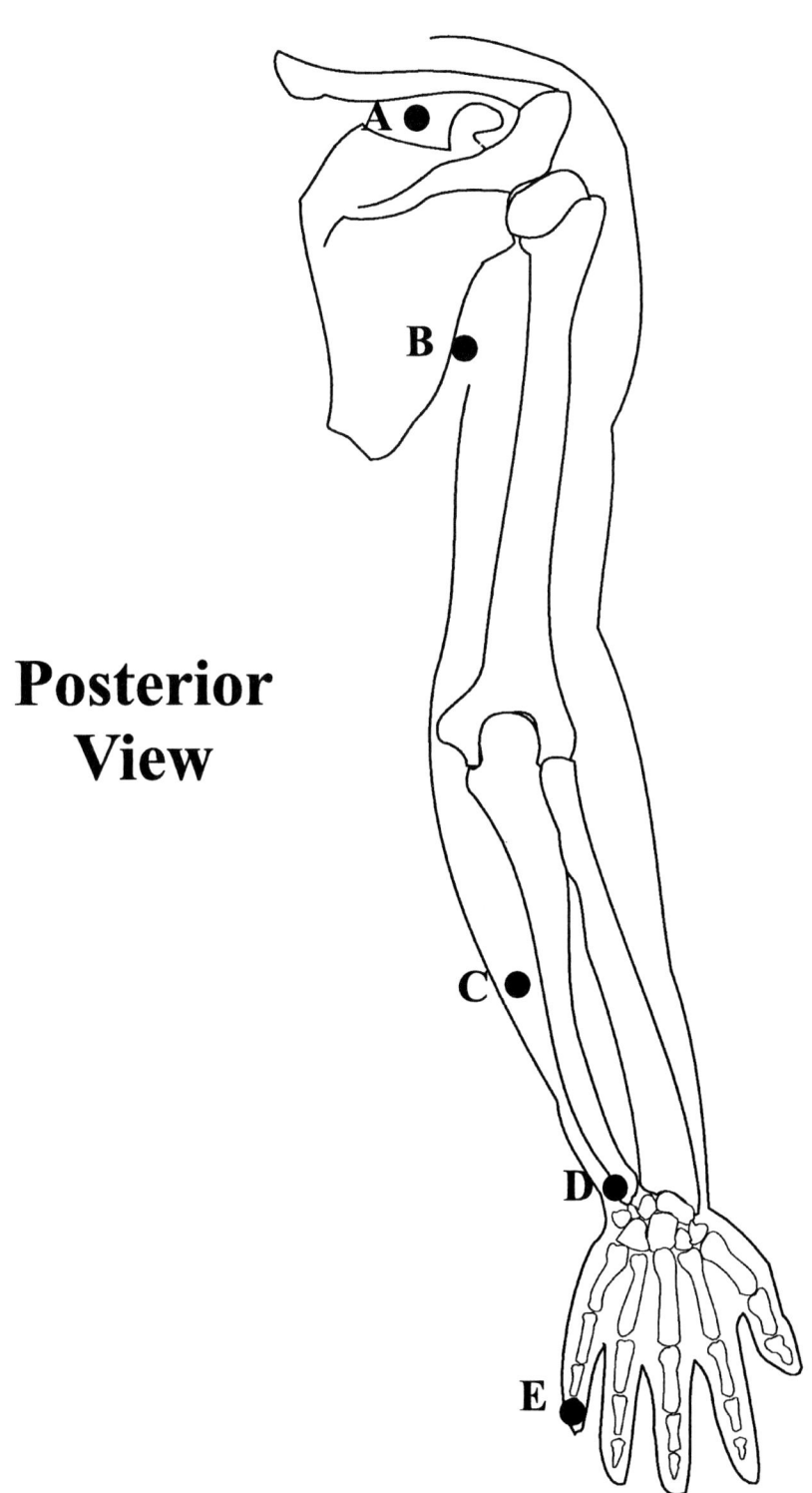

**Posterior
View**

480. Examine the diagram and determine which of these four acupoints is most proximal to acupoint B.

    a. E

    b. D

    c. C

    d. A

Answer: _____

Source: C-169, D-240

Bladder

481. The bladder channel originates at which anatomical structure?

    a. The bladder

    b. The tip of the small toe

    c. The inner canthus of the eye

    d. The outer canthus of the eye

Answer: _____

Source: C-73, D-251

482. Where does the bladder channel separate to connect with the kidney channel?

    a. On the lower leg, 3 *cun* directly superior to *Kun Lun* (Bl 60)

    b. On the lower leg, 7 *cun* directly superior to *Kun Lun* (Bl 60)

    c. Behind the ankle joint, in the depression between the prominence of the lateral malleolus and the Achilles tendon

    d. At the back of the knee, on the popliteal crease

Answer: _____

Source: C-188, D-316

483. Known as one of the "bone holes," which acupoint on the bladder channel is over the second posterior sacral foramen?

    a. *Shang Liao* (Bl 31)

    b. *Ci Liao* (Bl 32)

    c. *Zhong Liao* (Bl 33)

    d. *Xia Liao* (Bl 34)

Answer: _____

Source: C-182, D-293

484. Which of the following is the correct description for the location of *Yi She* (Bl 49)?

    a. 3 *cun* lateral to the midline, level with the lower border of the spinous process of the 3rd thoracic vertebra, on the spinal border of the scapula

    b. 3 *cun* lateral to the midline, level with the lower border of the spinous process of the 4th thoracic vertebra, on the spinal border of the scapula

    c. 3 *cun* lateral to the midline, level with the lower border of the spinous process of the 9th thoracic vertebra

    d. 3 *cun* lateral to the midline, level with the lower border of the spinous process of the 11th thoracic vertebra

Answer: _____

Source: C-186, D-308

485. Which acupoint is located 5.5 *cun* above the midpoint of the anterior hairline and 1.5 *cun* lateral to the midline?

    a. *Qu Cha* (Bl 4)

    b. *Cheng Guang* (Bl 6)

    c. *Luo Que* (Bl 8)

    d. *Tian Zhu* (Bl 10)

Answer: _____

Source: C-175, D-261

486. Which back transport point is located 1.5 *cun* lateral to the lower border of the spinous process of the 4th thoracic vertebra?

    a. *Fei Shu* (Bl 13)

    b. *Jue Yin Shu* (Bl 14)

    c. *Xin Shu* (Bl 15)

    d. *Du Shu* (Bl 16)

Answer: _____

Source: C-177, D-269

487. Which of the following is the correct description for the location of the blood master point?

    a. 1.5 *cun* lateral to the lower border of the spinous process of the 5th thoracic vertebra

    b. 1.5 *cun* lateral to the lower border of the spinous process of the 6th thoracic vertebra

    c. 1.5 *cun* lateral to the lower border of the spinous process of the 7th thoracic vertebra

    d. 1.5 *cun* lateral to the lower border of the spinous process of the 9th thoracic vertebra

Answer: _____

Source: C-178, D-272

Sources: C=CAM, D=Deadman, F=Flaws, S=Shanghai

488. The back transport of the gallbladder is located at the level of which vertebra?

    a. The 3rd thoracic vertebra

    b. The 9th thoracic vertebra

    c. The 10th thoracic vertebra

    d. The 1st lumbar vertebra

Answer: _____

Source: C-179, D-277

489. Which of the following is the correct description for the location of the source point of the bladder channel?

    a. On the lateral side of the foot, in the depression anterior and inferior to the tuberosity of the 5th metatarsal bone

    b. 3 *cun* directly above *Kun Lun* (Bl 60)

    c. In the depression directly below the malleolus

    d. On the lateral side of the foot, on the lower border of the cuboid bone

Answer: _____

Source: C-190, D-323

490. *Yu Zhen* (Bl 9) is closest to what prominent anatomical structure?

    a. The inner canthus of the eye

    b. The ear

    c. The 7th cervical vertebra

    d. The external occipital protuberance

Answer: _____

Source: C-176, D-262

For the following questions, refer to the diagram on the next page:

491. Acupoint A is in the center of the gluteal crease. Acupoint B is the uniting point on the bladder channel. What is the distance between acupoints A and B?

    a. 14 *cun*

    b. 16 *cun*

    c. 19 *cun*

    d. 21 *cun*

Answer: _____

Source: C-120, D-64

492. Acupoint C is *Wei Yang* (Bl 39). This acupoint is located medial to which tendon?

    a. The *semitendinosus*

    b. The *biceps femoris*

    c. The *peroneus longus*

    d. The *gastrocnemius*

Answer: _____

Source: C-184, D-298

493. Acupoint D is *Cheng Shan* (Bl 57). Acupoint E is located 1 *cun* inferior to acupoint D. Name acupoint E.

    a. *Cheng Jin* (Bl 56)

    b. The cleft point of the yang springing vessel

    c. The network point of the bladder channel

    d. The fire point of the bladder channel

Answer: _____

Source: C-188, D-316

494. If acupoint B is the uniting point of the bladder channel, and acupoint D is *Cheng Shan* (Bl 57), how many *cun* units are there between acupoints B and D?

    a. 6

    b. 7

    c. 8

    d. 12

Answer: _____

Source: C-188, D-316

Bladder 1

Posterior
View

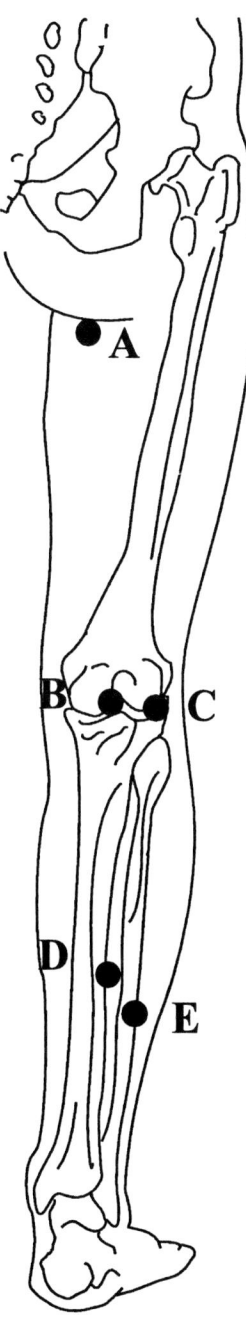

495. Which of these acupoints is the lower uniting point of the triple burner channel?

    a. A

    b. B

    c. C

    d. D

Answer: _____

Source: C-184, D-298

For the following questions, refer to the diagram on the next page:

496. Which of the following acupoints is the metal point on the bladder channel?

    a. A

    b. B

    c. D

    d. E

Answer: _____

Source: C-191, D-325

497. This acupoint is the river point on the bladder channel:

    a. A

    b. B

    c. D

    d. E

Answer: _____

Source: C-189, D-318

498. Which of these acupoints is the source point on the bladder channel?

    a. A

    b. B

    c. C

    d. D

Answer: _____

Source: C-190, D-323

499. If acupoint A is the well point on the bladder channel, and acupoint B is the next transport point in sequence. What is acupoint B?

    a. The fire point

    b. The earth point

    c. The water point

    d. The wood point

Answer: _____

Source: C-190, D-324

Sources: C=CAM, D=Deadman, F=Flaws, S=Shanghai

Bladder 2

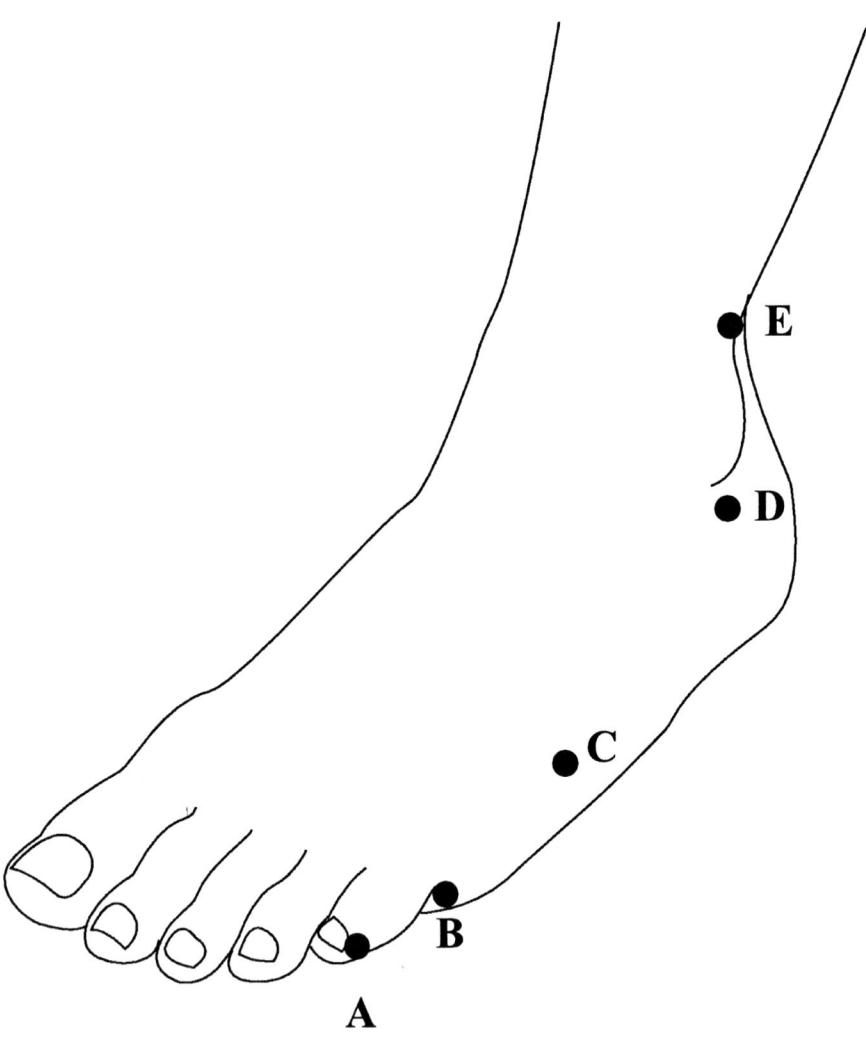

500. Which of these acupoints is the master point of the yang springing vessel?

      a. A

      b. B

      c. C

      d. D

Answer: _____

Source: C-190, D-320

Kidney

501. The kidney channel begins:

    a. In the right kidney

    b. Below the 12th "floating" rib

    c. Beneath the little toe

    d. On the leg near *San Yin Jiao* (Sp 6)

Answer: _____

Source: C-73, D-331

502. The kidney channel intersects which of the following bowels and viscera?

    a. Bladder

    b. Liver

    c. Heart

    d. All of the above

Answer: _____

Source: C-73-75, D-332

503. This acupoint on the kidney channel is the only well point not located on a finger or toe:

    a. *Shu Fu* (Ki 27)

    b. *Huang Zhu* (Ki 16)

    c. *Tai Xi* (Ki 3)

    d. *Yong Quan* (Ki 1)

Answer: _____

Source: C-191, D-336

504. Which of the following is the correct description for the location of the network point of the kidney channel?

    a. Anterior and inferior to the medial malleolus, in the depression on the lower border of the tuberosity of the navicular bone

    b. In the depression between the tip of the medial malleolus and Achilles tendon

    c. Posterior and inferior to the medial malleolus, in the depression anterior to the medial side of the the attachment of the Achilles tendon

    d. In the depression below the tip of the medial malleolus

Answer: _____

Source: C-192, D-342

505. How far is *Shui Quan* (Ki 5) from the stream point on the kidney channel?

    a. 1 *cun*

    b. 2 *cun*

    c. 3 *cun*

    d. 5 *cun*

Answer: _____

Source: C-192, D-343

506. Which anatomical structure is located closest to *Huang Zhu* (Ki 16)?

    a. The nipple

    b. The ankle

    c. The 11th "floating" rib

    d. The umbilicus

Answer: _____

Source: C-195, D-355

507. How many *cun* units are there between *Heng Gu* (Ki 11) and *Zhong Zhu* (Ki 15)?

    a. 2.1

    b. 3.5

    c. 4

    d. 5

Answer: _____

Source: C-194-195, D-351, 354

508. Which acupoint on the kidney channel is located in the fourth intercostal space, 2 *cun* lateral to the midline?

      a. *Bu Lang* (Ki 22)

      b. *Sheng Feng* (Ki 23)

      c. *Ling Xu* (Ki 24)

      d. *Shen Cang* (Ki 25)

Answer: _____

Source: C-197, D-360

509. Which acupoint on the kidney channel is located on the lower border of the clavicle?

      a. *Shu Fu* (Ki 27)

      b. *Yu Zhong* (Ki 26)

      c. *Shen Cang* (Ki 25)

      d. *Ling Xu* (Ki 24)

Answer: _____

Source: C-198, D-362

510. *Ying Gu* (Ki 10) is located between the *semitendinosus* and _____ tendons.

      a. *Gastrocnemius*

      b. *Semimembranosus*

      c. Achilles

      d. *Hallucis longus*

Answer: _____

Source: C-194, D-350

For the following questions, refer to the diagram on the next page:

511. Which of these acupoints is the source point of the kidney channel?

     a. B

     b. C

     c. D

     d. E

Answer: _____

Source: C-192, D-339

512. If acupoint D is *Tai Xi* (Ki 3), which of these acupoints is the cleft point of the yin springing vessel?

     a. E

     b. D

     c. C

     d. A

Answer: _____

Source: C-193, D-348

513. If acupoint B is the cleft point of the yin linking vessel, and acupoint D is *Tai Xi* (Ki 3), how far above D is B?

     a. 3 *cun*

     b. 4 *cun*

     c. 5 *cun*

     d. 8 *cun*

Answer: _____

Source: C-193, D-349

514. Which of these acupoints is the master point of the yin springing vessel?

     a. E

     b. D

     c. B

     d. A

Answer: _____

Source: C-193, D-344

Kidney

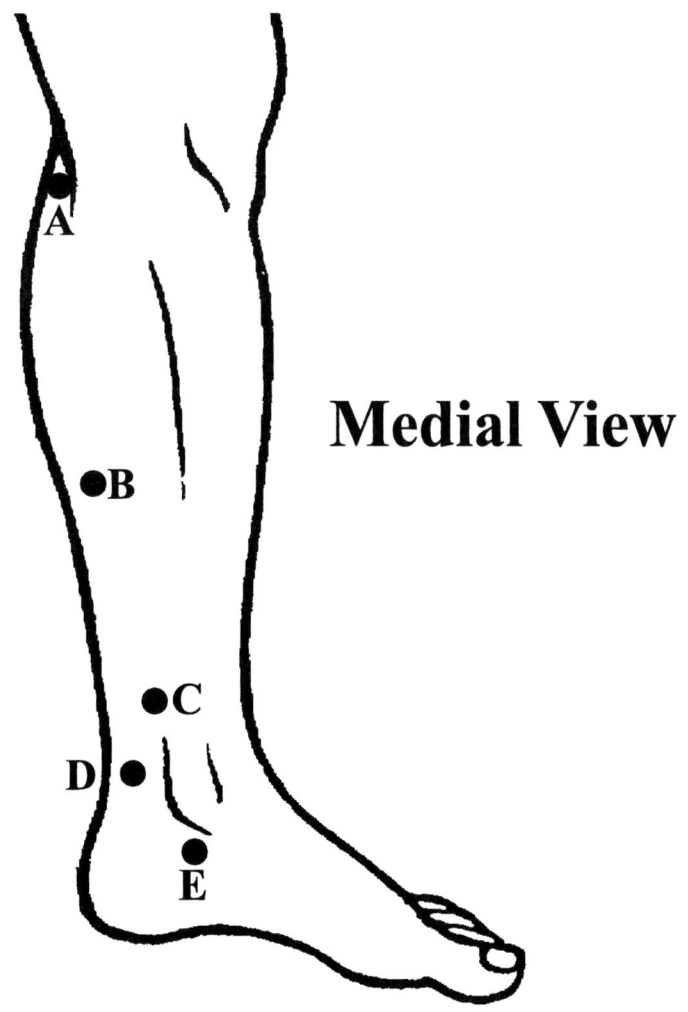

Medial View

Pericardium

515. The pericardium channel begins:

      a. In the 4th intercostal space, 1 *cun* lateral to the nipple

      b. In the heart

      c. In the center of the chest

      d. At the tip of the middle finger

Answer: _____

Source: C-77, D-367

516. Which of the following is the correct description for the location of the metal point of the pericardium channel?

      a. On the flexor aspect of the forearm, 5 *cun* proximal to *Da Ling* (Per 7)

      b. On the transverse cubital crease, at the ulnar side of the tendon of the *biceps brachii*

      c. 1 cun lateral to the nipple, in the 4th intercostal space

      d. On the flexor aspect of the forearm, 3 *cun* proximal to *Da Ling* (Per 7)

Answer: _____

Source: C-201, D-374

517. The cleft point of the pericardium channel lies between the tendons of the *palmaris longus* and the:

      a. *Extensor digitorum communis*

      b. *Flexor carpi radialis*

      c. *Extensor digiti minimi*

      d. *Flexor carpi ulnaris*

Answer: _____

Source: C-200, D-373

518. Which of the following acupoints is most distal to the uniting point of the pericardium channel?

      a. *Tian Quan* (Per 2)

      b. *Xi Men* (Per 4)

      c. *Nei Guan* (Per 6)

      d. *Lao Gong* (Per 8)

Answer: _____

Source: C-201, D-380

519. What is the distance between *Nei Guan* (Per 6) and *Qu Ze* (Per 3)?

   a. 6 *cun*

   b. 8 *cun*

   c. 10 *cun*

   d. 11 *cun*

Answer: _____

Source: C-200-201, D-372, 374

For the following questions, refer to the diagram on the next page:

520. If acupoint D is the uniting point of the pericardium channel and acupoint E is *Tian Quan* (Per 2), what is the distance between acupoints D and E?

    a. *5 cun*

    b. *7 cun*

    c. *8 cun*

    d. *9 cun*

Answer: _____

Source: C-199, 299, D-371, 372

521. Acupoint A is the fire point on the pericardium channel. What is the proper technique for locating it?

    a. Locate the point 3 *cun* below the crease of the wrist between the 2nd and 3rd metacarpal bones.

    b. Locate the point 5 *cun* below the tip of the middle finger.

    c. Measure the palm from medial to lateral edges, the point is in the center.

    d. When a soft fist is made, the point is located where the tip of the middle finger lands.

Answer: _____

Source: C-201, D-381

522. If acupoint B is the earth point and acupoint C is the master point of the yin linking vessel, what is the distance between acupoints B and C?

    a. 0.5 *cun*

    b. 1 *cun*

    c. 2 *cun*

    d. 2.5 *cun*

Answer: _____

Source: C-201, D-376, 378

523. If acupoint D is the water point on the pericardium channel, which acupoint is most proximal to acupoint D?

    a. A

    b. B

    c. C

    d. E

Answer: _____

Source: C-200, D-372

Sources: C=CAM, D=Deadman, F=Flaws, S=Shanghai

Pericardium

Anterior View

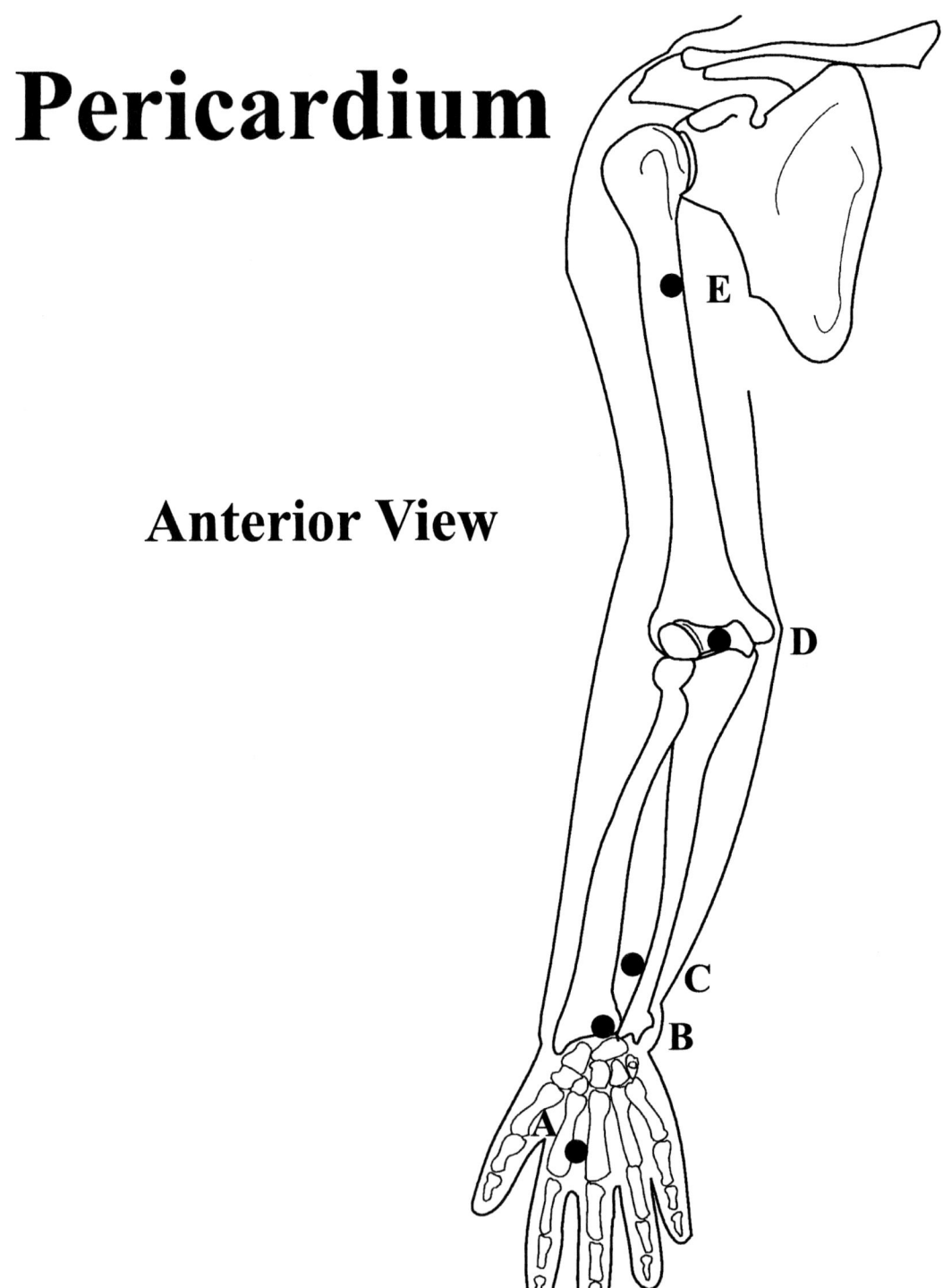

524. If acupoint B is the stream point on the pericardium channel, what is the warning associated with needling it?

    a. Deep puncture may damage the median nerve.

    b. Deep puncture may damage the ulnar nerve.

    c. Deep puncture may damage the radial artery.

    d. Deep puncture may damage the median artery.

Answer: _____

Source: C-201, D-378

Triple Burner

525. The triple burner channel has three distinct branches. One begins at the tip of the little finger, one separates at *Shan Zhong* (CV 17), and the third:

     a. Separates in the lower abdomen at *Zhong Ji* (CV 3)

     b. Separates at the outer canthus near *Tong Zi Liao* (GB 1)

     c. Separates in the stomach area at *Zhong Wan* (CV 12)

     d. Separates behind the ear near *Yi Feng* (TB 17)

Answer: _____

Source: C-77, D-388

526. Which of the following is the correct description for the location of the stream point of the triple burner channel?

     a. On the dorsal aspect of the ring finger, along the ulnar border of the nail

     b. On the dorsum of the wrist, at the level of the wrist joint

     c. Between the ring and little fingers, 0.5 *cun* proximal to the margin of the web

     d. On the dorsum of the hand, in the depression just proximal to the 4th and 5th metacarpo-phalangeal joints.

Answer: _____

Source: C-203, D-393

527. The master point of the yang linking vessel is how many *cun* units proximal to the transverse crease of the wrist?

     a. 1

     b. 2

     c. 3

     d. 5

Answer: _____

Source: C-203, D-396

528. The uniting point of the triple burner channel is 1 *cun* superior to what major anatomical structure?

     a. The tip of the humerus

     b. The tip of the olecranon

     c. The tip of the radius

     d. The tip of the ulna

Answer: _____

Source: C-205, D-402

529. What acupoint on the triple burner lies in the depression posterior and inferior to the lateral extremity of the acromion?

     a. *Qing Leng Yuan* (TB 11)

     b. *Xiao Luo* (TB 12)

     c. *Nao Hui* (TB 13)

     d. *Jian Liao* (TB 14)

Answer: _____

Source: C-206, D-405

530. Which acupoint on the triple burner is located directly above the ear apex?

     a. *Yi Feng* (TB 17)

     b. *Lu Xi* (TB 19)

     c. *Jiao Sun* (TB 20)

     d. *Er Men* (TB 21)

Answer: _____

Source: C-208, D-410

531. Which anatomical structure passes close to *Er He Liao* (TB 22)?

     a. The superficial temporal artery

     b. The auricular vein

     c. The outer canthus of the eye

     d. The lateral end of the eyebrow

Answer: _____

Source: C-208, D-411

532. Which acupoint on the triple burner channel is located on the posterior border of the *sternocleido-mastiodius* muscle?

      a. *Yi Feng* (TB 17)

      b. *Tian You* (TB 16)

      c. *Tian Liao* (TB 15)

      d. *Jian Liao* (TB 14)

Answer: _____

Source: C-206, D-407

533. How many *cun* units are between the fire point of the triple burner and *San Yang Luo* (TB 8)?

      a. 0.5

      b. 1

      c. 2

      d. 5

Answer: _____

Source: C-304, 305, D-401

534. Which of the acupoints on the triple burner channel lies closest to the eye?

      a. *Lu Xi* (TB 19)

      b. *Er Men* (TB 21)

      c. *Er He Liao* (TB 22)

      d. *Si Zhu Kong* (TB 23)

Answer: _____

Source: C-208, D-412

For the following questions, refer to the diagram on the next page:

535. If acupoint B is the cleft point on the triple burner channel, it is _____ the river point on the triple burner channel.

    a. Superior to

    b. Inferior to

    c. At the same level as

    d. 1 *cun* medial to

Answer: _____

Source: C-204, D-400

536. Acupoint A is *Si Du* (TB 9), and acupoint D is the source point on the triple burner channel. How many *cun* units are there between acupoints A and D?

    a. 9

    b. 7

    c. 5

    d. Cannot be determined

Answer: _____

Source: C-205, D-401

537. Which of these acupoints is the water point on the triple burner channel?

    a. B

    b. C

    c. D

    d. E

Answer: _____

Source: C-202, D-392

538. If acupoint C is the network point and acupoint D is the source point on the triple burner channel, how many *cun* units are there between C and D?

    a. 1.5

    b. 2

    c. 3

    d. Cannot be determined

Answer: _____

Source: C-203, D-395, 396

Triple Burner

Posterior View

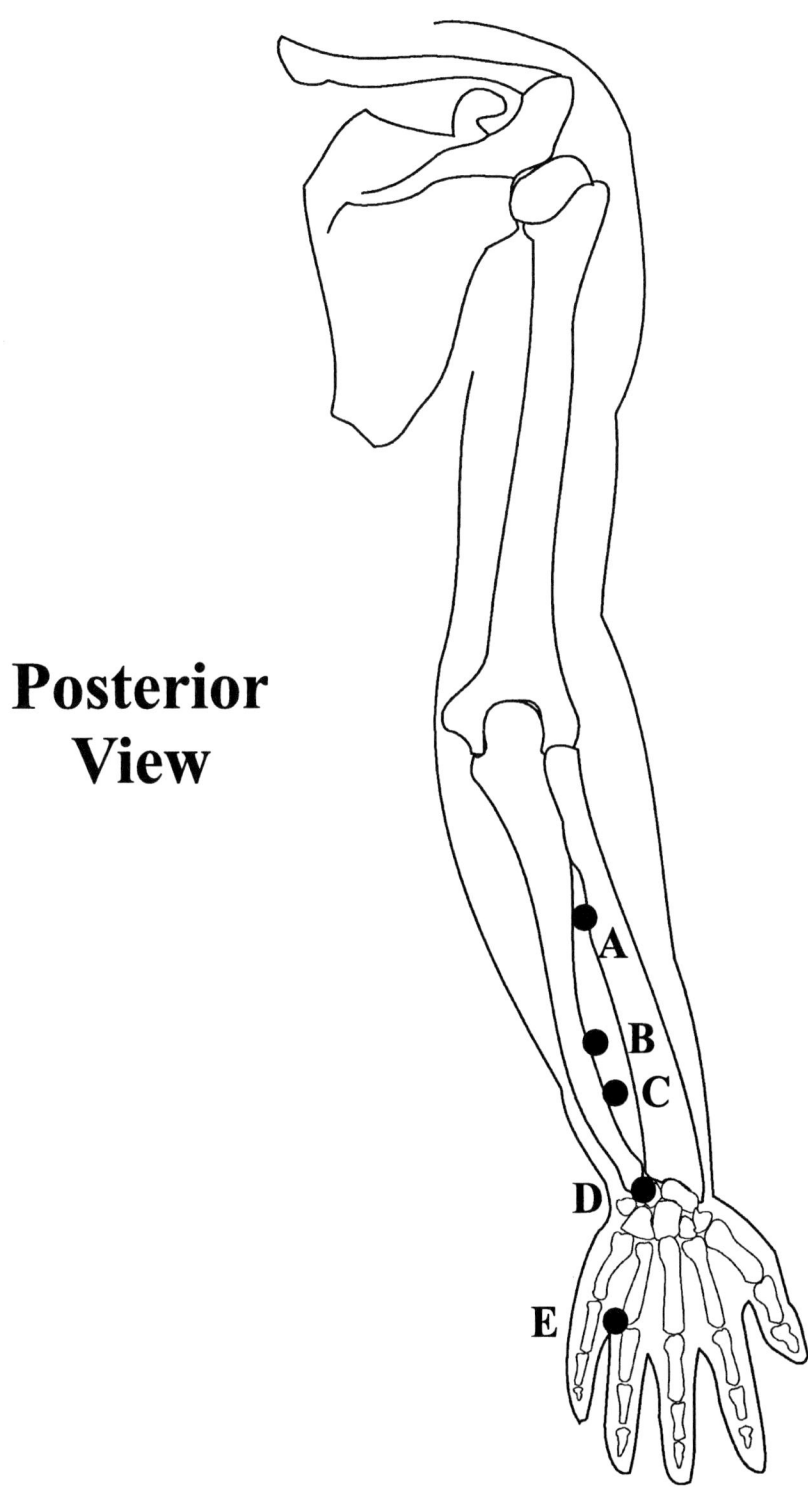

539. Which of the acupoints illustrated is most proximal to acupoint C?

    a. E

    b. D

    c. B

    d. A

Answer: _____

Source: C-204, D-400

Gallbladder

540. Two branches of the gallbladder channel end in the foot. One ends at the lateral side of the tip of the fourth toe, the other ends at:

    a. The bottom of the third toe

    b. The ankle near *Zhong Fen* (Liv 4)

    c. The hairy region of the big toe

    d. At *Guang Ming* (GB 37)

Answer: _____

Source: C-80, D-418

541. What technique is critical to properly locate and needle *Ting Lui* (GB 2)?

    a. The mouth should be closed and the jaws clenched to reveal the point

    b. The mouth should be open, but can be closed after the point is needled

    c. Locate and push the temporal artery out of the way

    d. Pull the ear back to tense the skin before needling the point

Answer: _____

Source: C-209, D-422

542. Which of the following is the correct description for the location of *Shuai Gu* (GB 8)?

    a. In the temporal region, within the hairline, 1 fingerbreath anterior to *Jiao Sun* (SJ 20)

    b. Superior to the apex of the auricle, 1.5 *cun* within the hairline

    c. Directly above the posterior border of the auricle, 2 *cun* within the hairline

    d. 2 *cun* anterior to *Fu Bai* (GB 10)

Answer: _____

Source: C-211, D-427

543. *Tou Lin Qi* (GB 15), *Mu Chuang* (GB 16), *Zheng Ying* (GB 17), and *Cheng Ling* (GB 18) are evenly spaced along the top of the head. How many *cun* units separate each of them?

    a. 0.5

    b. 1

    c. 1.5

    d. 3

Answer: _____

Source: C-212-213, D-432-435

544. What is the danger associated with needling *Feng Chi* (GB 20)?

   a. Deep needling may arouse too much yang qi.

   b. Deep needling may puncture the dorsal artery.

   c. Deep needling may puncture the *sternocleidomastoidius* muscle.

   d. Deep needling may puncture the spinal cord.

Answer: _____

Source: C-214, D-436

545. If *Jian Jing* (GB 21) is needled too deeply and perpendicularly, what can occur?

   a. The carotid artery may be punctured.

   b. The subclavian vein may be punctured.

   c. The upper lobe of the lung may be punctured.

   d. The acromion may be punctured.

Answer: _____

Source: C-214, D-438

546. At which intercostal space is the alarm point of the gallbladder channel located?

   a. 3rd

   b. 5th

   c. 7th

   d. 8th

Answer: _____

Source: C-215, D-441

547. Where is the alarm point of the kidney channel located?

   a. Directly below *Zhang Men* (Liv 13), level with the umbilicus

   b. Anterior and inferior to the free end of the 12th rib

   c. Directly below the nipple in the 7th intercostal space

   d. Below the axilla in the 4th intercostal space at the level of the nipple

Answer: _____

Source: C-215, D-442

548. *Huan Tiao* (GB 30) is located laterally _____ of the distance between the prominence of the greater trochanter and the hiatus of the sacrum.

    a. 1/3

    b. 1/4

    c. 3/4

    d. 1/5

Answer: _____

Source: C-217, D-446

549. *Feng Shi* (GB 31) is located how many *cun* units below the greater trochanter?

    a. 7

    b. 9

    c. 12

    d. 19

Answer: _____

Source: C-218, D-448

550. *Yang Ling Quan* (GB 34) is located anterior and inferior to what bony structure?

    a. The lateral epicondyle of the femur

    b. The head of the fibula

    c. The head of the tibia

    d. The base of the patella

Answer: _____

Source: C-218, D-450

551. The cleft point of the yang linking vessel is located how many *cun* units below the popliteal crease?

    a. 5

    b. 7

    c. 9

    d. 12

Answer: _____

Source: C-219, D-453

Sources: C=CAM, D=Deadman, F=Flaws, S=Shanghai

552. The master point of marrow is located between the tendons of the:

    a. *Peroneus longus* and *brevis*

    b. *Semimembranosus* and *tendinosus*

    c. Posterior and anterior *tibialis*

    d. *Extensor digiti minimi*

Answer: _____

Source: C-220, D-457

553. *Zu Ling Qi* (GB 41) is needled _____ to the tendon of the *extensor digiti minimi.*

    a. Medial

    b. Lateral

    c. Superior

    d. Anterior

Answer: _____

Source: C-230, D-460

554. Which acupoint on the gallbladder channel is located in the depression anterior and inferior to the lateral malleolus?

    a. The wood point

    b. The spring point

    c. The master point of marrow

    d. The source point

Answer: _____

Source: C-220, D-458

For the following questions, refer to the diagram on the next page:

555. The gallbladder channel has two cleft points on it. One is *Yang Jiao* (GB 35), the other is acupoint C, which is:

    a. *Yang Ling Quan* (GB 34)

    b. *Wai Qiu* (GB 36)

    c. *Guang Ming* (GB 37)

    d. *Yang Fu* (GB 38)

Answer: _____

Source: C-219, D-453

556. Acupoint B is located 7 *cun* above acupoint D, which is the source point on the gallbladder channel. What other point on the gallbladder channel is located 7 *cun* above the source point?

    a. The earth point

    b. The network point

    c. The cleft point of the yang linking vessel

    d. The river point

Answer: _____

Source: C-219, D-452

557. Which of these acupoints is the wood point on the gallbladder channel?

    a. B

    b. C

    c. D

    d. E

Answer: _____

Source: C-220, D-460

558. Acupoint C is the fire point on the gallbladder channel. If acupoint D is the source point, how many *cun* units separate C and D?

    a. 3

    b. 4

    c. 5

    d. 7

Answer: _____

Source: C-219, 220, D-455

Gallbladder

**Lateral
View**

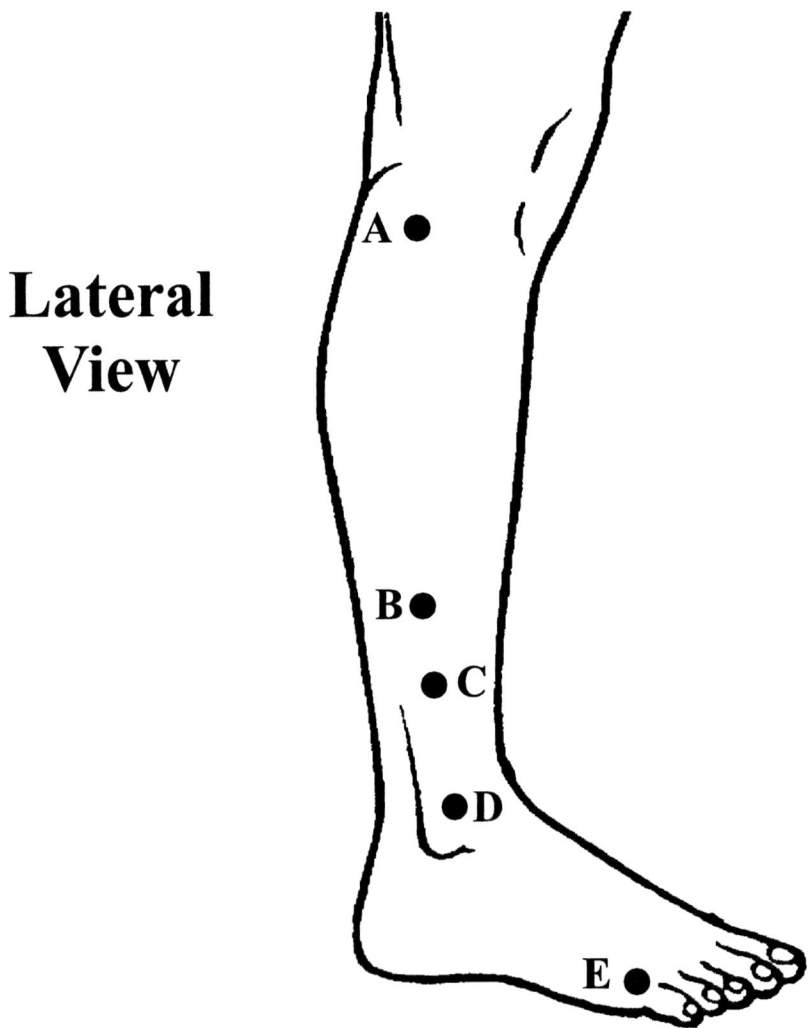

559. Which of these acupoints is the master point of the sinews?

     a. A

     b. B

     c. D

     d. E

Answer: _____

Source: C-218, D-450

Liver

560. Where does the liver channel intersect the spleen channel?

    a. At *Da Dun* (Liv 1)

    b. At *Tai Chong* (Liv 3)

    c. At *Li Gou* (Liv 5)

    d. At *San Yin Jiao* (Sp 6)

Answer: _____

Source: C-69, D-469

561. The liver channel of foot *jue yin* connects with the liver, gallbladder, lung, and:

    a. Spleen

    b. Heart

    c. Stomach

    d. Triple burner

Answer: _____

Source: C-81, D-470

562. Which of the following is the correct description for the location of the fire point on the liver channel?

    a. On the dorsum of the foot, between the first and second toes, proximal to the margin of the web at the junction of the red and white skin

    b. On the dorsum of the foot, in the depression distal to the junction of the first and second metatarsal bones

    c. On the dorsum of the foot, between the second and third toes, proximal to the margin of the web at the junction of the red and white skin

    d. On the dorsum of the foot, between the third and fourth toes, proximal to the margin of the web at the junction of the red and white skin

Answer: _____

Source: C-221-222, D-474

563. The network point on the liver channel is located how many *cun* above the tip of the medial malleolus?

    a. 3

    b. 5

    c. 9

    d. 12

Answer: _____

Source: C-223, D-482

564. *Xi Guan* (Liv 7) is located 1 *cun* posterior to which acupoint located near the knee?

    a. *Yin Gu* (Ki 10)

    b. *Yang Ling Quan* (GB 34)

    c. *Yin Ling Quan* (Sp 9)

    d. *Qu Quan* (Liv 8)

Answer: _____

Source: C-223, D-484

565. Which acupoint on the liver channel is located 2 *cun* directly below *Qi Chong* (St 30) and on the lateral border of the *adductus longus* muscle?

    a. *Yin Bao* (Liv 9)

    b. *Zu Wu Li* (Liv 10)

    c. *Yin Lian* (Liv 11)

    d. *Ji Mai* (Liv 12)

Answer: _____

Source: C-225, D-487

566. The alarm point of the spleen is found near which rib?

    a. 4th

    b. 6th

    c. 11th

    d. 12th

Answer: _____

Source: C-226, D-488

567. What is the caution associated with needling the alarm point of the liver?

    a. Deep, perpendicular insertion carries the risk of penetrating the liver.

    b. Deep, perpendicular insertion carries the risk of penetrating the spleen.

    c. Deep, perpendicular insertion carries the risk of penetrating the peritoneum.

    d. Deep, perpendicular insertion carries the risk of penetrating the lung.

Answer: _____

Source: C-226, D-490

568. The water point on the liver channel is located in the depression between which two tendons?

    a. The *sartorius* and *gracilis*

    b. The *peroneus longus* and *brevis*

    c. The *gastrocnemius* and Achilles

    d. The *semimembranosus* and *semitendinosus*

Answer: _____

Source: C-223, D-485

569. How many *cun* units are there between the cleft and network points on the liver channel?

    a. 1

    b. 2

    c. 3

    d. 5

Answer: _____

Source: C-223, D-482, 483

For the following questions, refer to the diagram on the next page:

570. Which of these acupoints is most distal to acupoint B?

    a. E

    b. C

    c. A

    d. Cannot be determined

571. If acupoint D is the cleft point of the liver channel, how many *cun* units are there between D and the tip of the medial malleolus?

    a. 7

    b. 8

    c. 9

    d. 12

Answer: _____

Source: C-223-224, D-483, 485

572. If acupoint C is the river point on the liver channel, what bony landmark is it close to?

    a. The bony tip of the lateral malleolus

    b. The bony tip of the medial malleolus

    c. The bony tip of the fibula

    d. The bony tip of the femur

Answer: _____

Source: C-222, D-480

573. One of these points on the liver channel is the source point. Which is it?

    a. E

    b. D

    c. B

    d. A

Answer: _____

Source: C-222, D-477

Liver

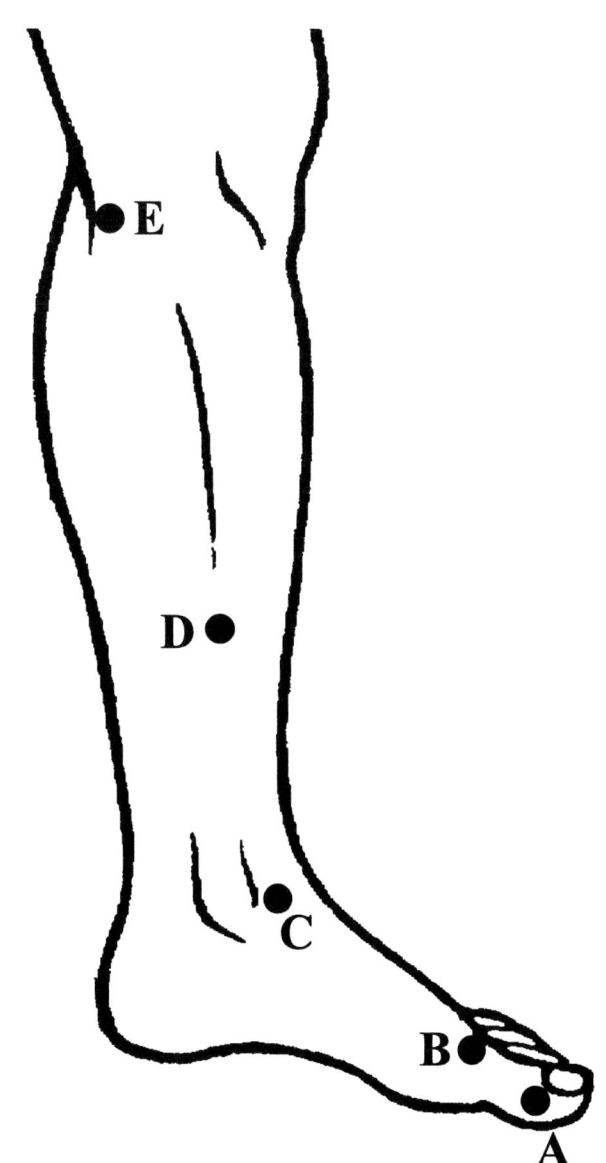

Medial
View

574. Acupoint A is the wood point on the liver channel. Approximately how many *cun* units is it located from the base of the nail of the great toe?

     a. 0.1

     b. 1

     c. 1.5

     d. None of the above

Answer: _____

Source: C-221, D-473

Conception Vessel

575. Where does the conception vessel begin?

    a. At the perineum, midway between the anus and scrotum or anus and posterior labial commissure.

    b. On the midline, midway between the coccyx and the anus

    c. In the lower abdomen

    d. In the middle burner near *Zhong Wan* (CV 12)

Answer: _____

Source: C-83, D-495

576. The conception vessel has a network channel that branches off from it. Where does this network channel begin?

    a. In the lower abdomen

    b. In the center of the sternum near *Shan Zhong* (CV 17).

    c. At the throat near *Tian Tu* (CV 22).

    d. In the upper burner near *Jiu Wei* (CV 15).

Answer: _____

Source: C-239, D-496

577. Which acupoint on the conception vessel is located 3 *cun* inferior to the umbilicus?

    a. *Qu Gu* (CV 2)

    b. *Zhong Ji* (CV 3)

    c. *Guan Yuan* (CV 4)

    d. *Shi Men* (CV 5)

Answer: _____

Source: C-237, D-501

578. What is the caution associated with needling *Qi Hai* (CV 6)?

    a. Deep needling may puncture the aorta.

    b. Deep needling may puncture the vena cava.

    c. Deep needling may penetrate the peritoneum.

    d. Deep needling may penetrate the bladder.

Answer: _____

Source: C-237, D-504

579. *Qi Hai* (CV 6) is located how many *cun* units from the navel?

    a. 0.5 *cun* inferior

    b. 1 *cun* superior

    c. 1.5 *cun* inferior

    d. 2 *cun* superior

Answer: _____

Source: C-237, D-504

580. What is the caution associated with *Shen Que* (CV 8)?

    a. Needling of this acupoint is forbidden.

    b. Moxibustion on this acupoint is forbidden.

    c. Needling and moxibustion on this acupoint are forbidden.

    d. No cautions are associated with this point.

Answer: _____

Source: C-238, D-507

581. How many *cun* units are between the alarm point of the small intestine channel and the alarm point of the stomach channel?

    a. 3

    b. 5

    c. 7

    d. 12

Answer: _____

Source: C-237-238, D-501, 511

582. Which of the following is the correct description for the location of the alarm point of the heart channel?

    a. On the anterior midline of the abdomen, at the sternocostal angle

    b. On the anterior midline of the abdomen, at the level of the 4th intercostal space

    c. On the anterior midline of the abdomen, 5 *cun* above the umbilicus

    d. On the anterior midline of the abdomen, 6 *cun* above the umbilicus

Answer: _____

Source: C-239, D-514

583. Both the alarm point of the pericardium and *Hua Gai* (CV 20) are located level with intercostal spaces. How many intercostal spaces separate them?

    a. 1

    b. 2

    c. 3

    d. 4

Answer: _____

Source: C-239-240, D-517, 520

584. What is the needling technique required for proper puncture of *Tian Tu* (CV 22)?

    a. Push in perpendicularly to a depth of 1.5 *cun,* use strong stimulation on the needle.

    b. Needle obliquely and upwards to a depth of 0.5 *cun* along the larynx.

    c. Push in perpendiculary to a depth of .2 *cun*, then guide the needle downward along the posterior border of the manubrium.

    d. No needling is allowed, only moxibustion.

Answer: _____

Source: C-240, D-522

For the following questions, refer to the diagram on the next page:

585. From its location on the drawing, identify acupoint A.

    a. *Ju Que* (CV 14)

    b. *Jiu Wei* (CV 15)

    c. *Zhong Ting* (CV 16)

    d. *Shan Zhong* (CV 17)

Answer: _____

Source: C-239, D-517

586. If acupoint B is the alarm point of the stomach and acupoint C is *Shi Fen* (CV 9), how many *cun* are there between acupoints B and C?

    a. 2

    b. 3

    c. 4

    d. 5

Answer: _____

Source: C-238, D-508, 511

587. Acupoint D is the alarm point of the triple burner channel. How many *cun* units is this point located inferior to the umbilicus?

    a. 1.5

    b. 2

    c. 3

    d. 4

Answer: _____

Source: C-237, D-503

588. Which of these acupoints is the alarm point of the bladder channel?

    a. A

    b. C

    c. E

    d. None of the above

Answer: _____

Source: C-236, D-499

Conception Vessel

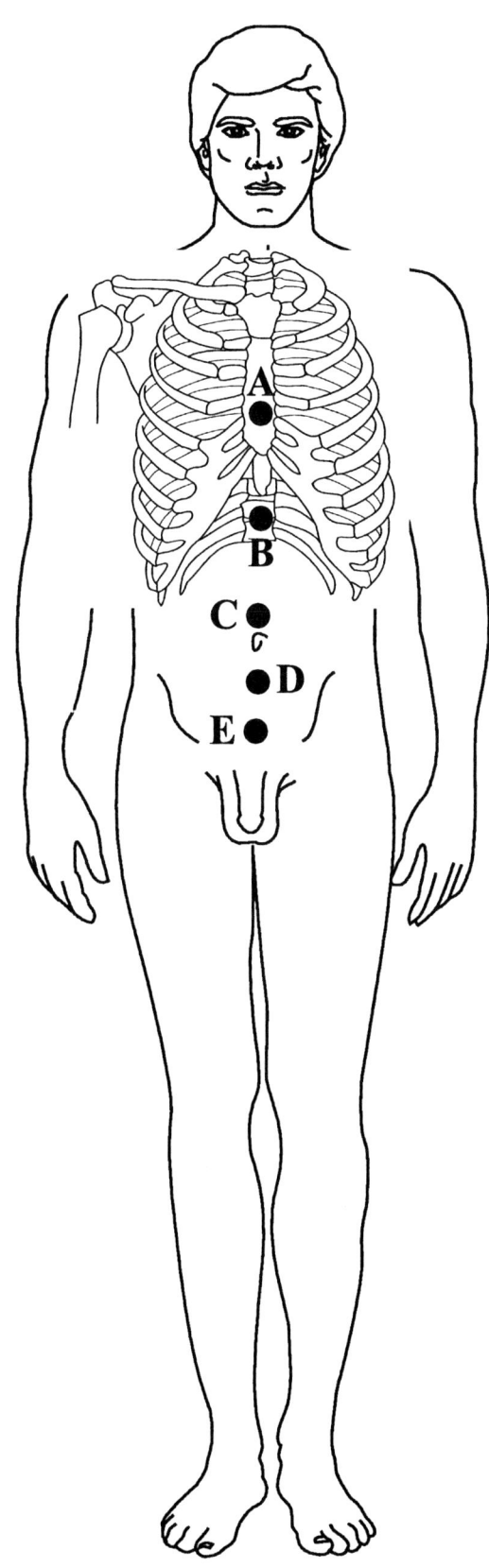

589. Which of these acupoints is located closest to the network point of the conception vessel?

    a. A

    b. C

    c. D

    d. E

Answer: _____

Source: C-239, D-515

Governing Vessel

590. The most superior of the branches of the governing vessel emerges at:

    a. The perineum at *Chang Qiang* (GV 1)

    b. The spine at *Ming Men* (GV 4)

    c. The eye at *Jing Ming* (Bl 1)

    d. The base of the skull at *Ya Men* (GV 15)

Answer: _____

Source: C-83, D-530

591. Which acupoint on the governing vessel is located at the hiatus of the sacrum?

    a. *Chang Qiang* (GV 1)

    b. *Yao Shu* (GV 2)

    c. *Yao Yang Guan* (GV 3)

    d. None of the above

Answer: _____

Source: C-227, D-535

592. Which acupoint on the governing vessel is located below the spinous process of the 7th thoracic vertebra?

    a. *Zhong Shu* (GV 7)

    b. *Jin Suo* (GV 8)

    c. *Zhi Yang* (GV 9)

    d. *Ling Tai* (GV 10)

Answer: _____

Source: C-230, D-540

593. How many cervical vertebrae are located between *Tao Dao* (GV 11) and *Feng Du* (CV 16)?

    a. 12

    b. 9

    c. 7

    d. 5

Answer: _____

Source: C-231-232, D-542, 548

594. "Below the spinous process of the seventh cervical vertebra, approximately at the level of the shoulders." This describes the location of which acupoint on the governing vessel?

  a. *Shen Zhu* (GV 12)

  b. *Da Zhui* (GV 14)

  c. *Ya Men* (GV 15)

  d. *Feng Du* (GV 16)

Answer: _____

Source: C-231, D-545

595. Which of the following is the correct description for the location of the network point of the governing vessel?

  a. Midway between the tip of the coccyx and anus

  b. Below the spinous process of the 1st lumbar vertebra

  c. In the depression below the spinous process of the 1st cervical vertebra

  d. Below the spinous process of the 2nd lumbar vertebra

Answer: _____

Source: C-227, D-534

596. Where is the lower sea of marrow acupoint located?

  a. Between the tip of the coccyx and anus

  b. Below the spinous process of the 2nd lumbar vertebra

  c. In the depression below the external occipital protuberance

  d. On the top of the head, 8 *cun* superior to the glabella

Answer: _____

Source: C-232, D-548

597. Which acupoint on the governing vessel is located 1 *cun* directly above the midpoint of the anterior hairline?

  a. *Xin Hui* (GV 22)

  b. *Shang Xing* (GV 23)

  c. *Shen Ting* (GV 24)

  d. *Su Liao* (GV 25)

Answer: _____

Source: C-234, D-556

598. *Su Liao* (GV 25) is located at which major anatomical structure?

    a. The center of the glabella

    b. The midpoint of the nape of the neck

    c. The tip of the nose

    d. The center of the upper lip

Answer: _____

Source: C-234, D-558

599. What is the caution associated with needling *Feng Fu* (GV 16)?

    a. No needling permitted on this point, moxibustion only.

    b. Deep puncture may penetrate the spinal canal.

    c. Deep, superior insertion toward the medullary bulb is required.

    d. Should not be needled on patients younger than 20 years of age.

Answer: _____

Source: C-232, D-548

For the following questions, refer to the diagram on the next page:

600. Acupoint A is *5.5 cun* directly above the midpoint of the posterior hairline. Name this acupoint.

  a. *Ya Men* (GV 15)

  b. *Feng Fu* (GV 16)

  c. *Qiang Jian* (GV 18)

  d. *Hou Ding* (GV 19)

Answer: _____

Source: C-233, D-551

601. If acupoint D is *Ming Men* (GV 4), then what is acupoint C?

  a. *Ji Zhong* (GV 6)

  b. *Jin Suo* (GV 8)

  c. *Zhi Yang* (GV 9)

  d. *Shen Dao* (GV 11)

Answer: _____

Source: C-230, D-540

602. Which of these acupoints is located at the sacrococcygeal hiatus?

  a. A

  b. C

  c. D

  d. E

Answer: _____

Source: C-227, D-535

603. If acupoint B is *Da Zhui* (GV 14) and acupoint D is *Ming Men* (GV 4), how many thoracic vertebrae are there between these two acupoints?

  a. 14

  b. 12

  c. 3

  d. Cannot be determined

Answer: _____

Source: C-228, 231, D-536, 545

Governing Vessel

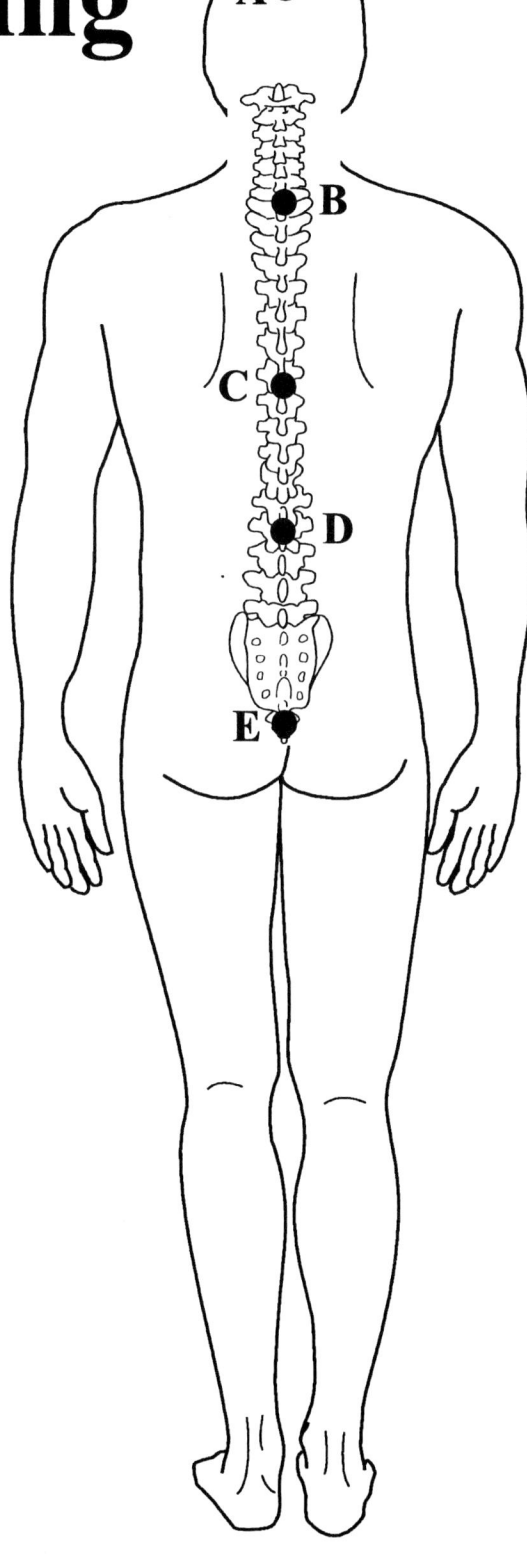

604. Acupoint C lies in which vertebral region?

   a. The cervical

   b. The thoracic

   c. The lumbar

   d. The sacral

Answer: _____

Source: C-230, D-540

Non-channel Points

605. Which non-channel acupoint is located midway between the medial ends of the two eyebrows?

    a. *Yin Tang* (M-HN-3)

    b. *Yu Yao* (M-HN-6)

    c. *Qiu Hou* (M-HN-8)

    d. *Tai Yang* (M-HN-9)

Answer: _____

Source: C-242, D-565

606. Which of these non-channel acupoints lies closest to the tip of the ear?

    a. *An Mian* (N-HN-54)

    b. *Bi Tong* (M-HN-14)

    c. *Er Jian* (M-HN-10)

    d. *Bai Liao* (M-HN-30)

Answer: _____

Source: C-242, D-558

607. Two non-channel acupoints can be found on either side of the frenulum of the tongue. One is *Jin Jin*, the other is _____.

    a. *Si Shen Cong* (M-HN-1)

    b. *Jia Cheng Jiang* (M-HN-18)

    c. *Yi Ming* (M-HN-13)

    d. *Yu Ye* (M-HN-20)

Answer: _____

Source: C-244, D-570

608. Which non-channel acupoints is found 0.5 *cun* lateral to *Da Zhui* (GV 14)?

    a. *Ding Chuan* (M-BW-1)

    b. *Yao Yan* (M-BW-24)

    c. *Wei Guan Xia Shu* (M-BW-12)

    d. *Hua Tuo Jia Ji* (M-BW-35)

Answer: _____

Source: C-245, D-571

609. These two non-channel acupoints are located at the same level on the abdomen as *Zhong Ji* (CV 3):

      a. *San Jiao Jiu* (M-CA-23)

      b. *Zi Gong Xue* (M-CA-18)

      c. *Ti Tuo* (N-CA-4)

      d. *Qi Men* (M-CA-15)

Answer: _____

Source: C-248, D-575

610. These four non-channel acupoints are found on the proximal interphalangeal joints of the index, middle, ring, and little fingers:

      a. *Shi Xuan* (M-UE-1)

      b. *Si Feng* (M-UE-9)

      c. *Ba Xie* (M-UE-22)

      d. *Yao Tong Xue* (N-UE-19)

Answer: _____

Source: C-577, D-249

611. Which non-channel acupoint is found on the dorsum of the hand in the depression just proximal to the 2nd and 3rd metacarpophalangeal joints?

      a. *Ba Xie* (M-UE-22)

      b. *Yao Tong Xue* (N-UE-19)

      c. *Shi Xuan* (M-UE-1)

      d. *Luo Zhen* (M-UE-24)

Answer: _____

Source: C-250, D-579

612. Which non-channel acupoint is located between the end of the anterior axillary fold and *Jian Yu* (LI 15)?

      a. *Zhou Jian* (M-UE-46)

      b. *Er Bai* (M-UE-29)

      c. *Jian Qian* (M-UE-48)

      d. *Tai Jian* (N-UE-11)

Answer: _____

Source: C-249, D-581

613. This set of non-channel acupoints is located in the eyes of the knee:

     a. *Bai Chong Wo* (M-LE-34)

     b. *He Ding* (M-LE-27)

     c. *Xi Yan* (MN-LE-16)

     d. *Zu Yi Cong* (N-LE-16)

Answer: _____

Source: C-252, D-583

614. Known as the "Appendix Point," this non-channel acupoint can be found 2 *cun* distal to *Zu San Li* (St 36):

     a. *Xi Yan* (MN-LE-16)

     b. *Lan Wei Xue* (M-LE-13)

     c. *Dan Nang Xue* (M-LE-23)

     d. *Bai Chong Wo* (M-LE-34)

Answer: _____

Source: C-252, D-583

Ear Acupuncture

615. The ear acupoint for treating patterns involving the knee is located:

   a. On the scapha

   b. On the tragus

   c. On the inferior crus of the antehelix

   d. On the superior crus of the antehelix

Answer: _____

Source: C-537, S-481

616. "Slightly above the parting of the two crura of the antehelix, in the triangular fossa." This is the location of which ear acupoint?

   a. Neurogate (*Shen Men)*

   b. Prostate

   c. Uterus

   d. Spleen

Answer: _____

Source: C-538, S-485

617. Which acupoint on the ear is located in the cymba concha above the small intestine point?

   a. Kidney

   b. Liver

   c. Spleen

   d. Lung

Answer: _____

Source: C-540, S-487

618. These two ear acupoints are found above and below the heart point:

   a. Kidney

   b. Ovary

   c. Lung

   d. Eye

Answer: _____

Source: C-541, S-489

619. The groove for lowering blood pressure is located:

    a. Near the tragus

    b. Above the cymba concha

    c. Near the triangular fossa

    d. On the back of the ear

Answer: _____

Source: C-542, S-490

620. The ear acupoint for treating patterns involving the shoulder is located:

    a. On the helix crus

    b. On the scapha

    c. On the antetragus

    d. On the cavum concha

Answer: _____

Source: C-536, S-480

621. This acupoint, which treats patterns involving the ischium and sciatic nerve, is located on what ear structure?

    a. The antetragus

    b. The cymba concha

    c. The inferior helix crus of the antehelix

    d. The scapha

Answer: _____

Source: C-537, S-482

622. "At the tip of the lower tubercle on the border of the tragus." This is a description of which ear acupoint?

    a. Throat

    b. Adrenal

    c. Large Intestine

    d. Testicles

Answer: _____

Source: C-538, S-483

623. This ear acupoint, which stops wheezing and is used for asthma, is located:

    a. At the tip of the antetragus

    b. On the cavum concha

    c. On the helix crus

    d. On the scapha

Answer: _____

Source: C-538, S-484

624. In what region of the ear is the acupoint for treating patterns of the spleen found?

    a. The cymba concha

    b. The cavum concha

    c. The antetragus

    d. The triangular fossa

Answer: _____

Source: C-541, S-488

For the following questions, refer to the diagram on the next page:

625. Which of the acupoints would be used to treat patterns involving the heart?

    a. E

    b. D

    c. C

    d. B

Answer: _____

Source: C-540, S-488

626. Which of these ear acupoints is *Shen Men* or Neurogate?

    a. A

    b. B

    c. C

    d. E

Answer: _____

Source: C-537, S-485

627. Which of these acupoints would be used to treat pain of the elbow?

    a. E

    b. D

    c. C

    d. B

Answer: _____

Source: C-536, S-480

628. Which of these ear acupoints is the Brain point?

    a. B

    b. C

    c. D

    d. E

Answer: _____

Source: C-539, S-484

Ear

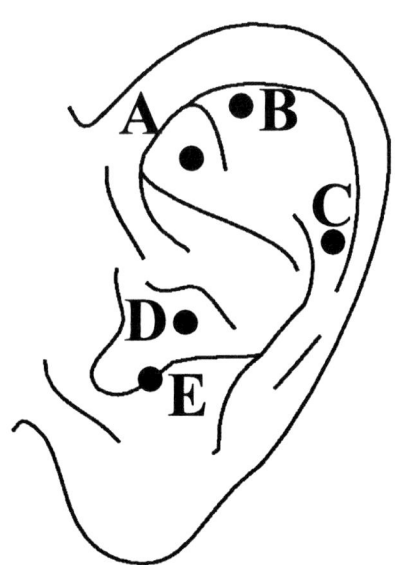

629. Which of these acupoints is located on the superior antehelix crus?

    a. A

    b. B

    c. C

    d. E

Answer: _____

Source: C-536, S-481

Mixed Channels

630. All of the following acupoints are located in the eyebrow *except*:

    a. *Qiu Hou* (M-HN-8)

    b. *Zan Zhu* (Bl 2)

    c. *Yu Yao* (M-HN-6)

    d. *Si Zhu Kong* (TB 23)

Answer: _____

Source: C-243, D-566

631. Which of the following acupoints is on the same body level as *Ya Men* (GV 15)?

    a. *Feng Chi* (GB 20)

    b. *Nao Gong* (GB 19)

    c. *Tian Zhu* (Bl 10)

    d. *Yu Zhen* (Bl 9)

Answer: _____

Source: C-176, 231, D-263, 546

632. All of the following acupoints are 0.5 *cun* units within the hairline *except*:

    a. *Tou Lin Qi* (GB 15)

    b. *Shang Xing* (GV 23)

    c. *Mei Chong* (Bl 3)

    d. *Qu Chai* (Bl 4)

Answer: _____

Source: C-234, D-556

633. Which of the following acupoints is *not* on a line level with the nipple?

    a. *Shan Zhong* (CV 17)

    b. *Tian Chi* (Per 1)

    c. *Ru Zhong* (St 17)

    d. *Bu Lang* (Ki 22)

Answer: _____

Source: C-187, D-359

634. All of the following acupoints are level with the tip of the laryngeal prominence *except*:

    a. *Ren Ying* (St 9)

    b. *Tian You* (TB 16)

    c. *Fu Tu* (LI 18)

    d. *Yian Chiang* (SI 16)

Answer: _____

Source: C-206, D-407

635. Which of the following acupoints is *not* located at the nose?

    a. *Ying Xiang* (LI 20)

    b. *Su Liao* (GV 25)

    c. *Cheng Jiang* (CV 24)

    d. *Bi Tong* (M-HN-14)

Answer: _____

Source: C-241, D-524

636. Which of the following ear points is most inferior?

    a. *Ting Hui* (GB 2)

    b. *Ting Gong* (SI 19)

    c. *Er Men* (TB 21)

    d. *Wang Gu* (GB 12)

Answer: _____

Source: C-211, D-430

637. Which of the following acupoints is *not* on a line with *Shen Que* (CV 8)?

    a. *Zhong Zhu* (Ki 15)

    b. *Tian Shu* (St 25)

    c. *Da Heng* (Sp 15)

    d. *Dai Mai* (GB 26)

Answer: _____

Source: C-195, D-354

638. At the level of *Jian Li* (CV 11), how many *cun* separate the spleen channel and the kidney channel?

    a. 2

    b. 2.5

    c. 3

    d. 3.5

Answer: _____

Source: C-161, 195, 238, D-201, 356, 510

639. Which of the following acupoints is most medial?

    a. *Qu Chi* (LI 11)

    b. *Shao Hai* (Ht 3)

    c. *Chi Ze* (Lu 5)

    d. *Qu Ze* (Per 3)

Answer: _____

Source: C-164, D-214

For the following questions, refer to the diagram on the next page:

640. Which of these acupoints is the uniting point of the spleen channel?

    a. A

    b. B

    c. E

    d. G

Answer: _____

Source: C-159, D-194

641. Which of these acupoints is the earth point on an earth channel?

    a. A

    b. C

    c. D

    d. E

Answer: _____

Source: C-154, D-158

642. Which of these acupoints is the network point on the stomach channel?

    a. A

    b. C

    c. D

    d. E

Answer: _____

Source: C-155, D-165

643. This acupoint is where the kidney, spleen, and liver channels intersect:

    a. G

    b. F

    c. E

    d. C

Answer: _____

Source: C-158, D-189

Sources: C=CAM, D=Deadman, F=Flaws, S=Shanghai

Mixed Channels 1

Anterior View

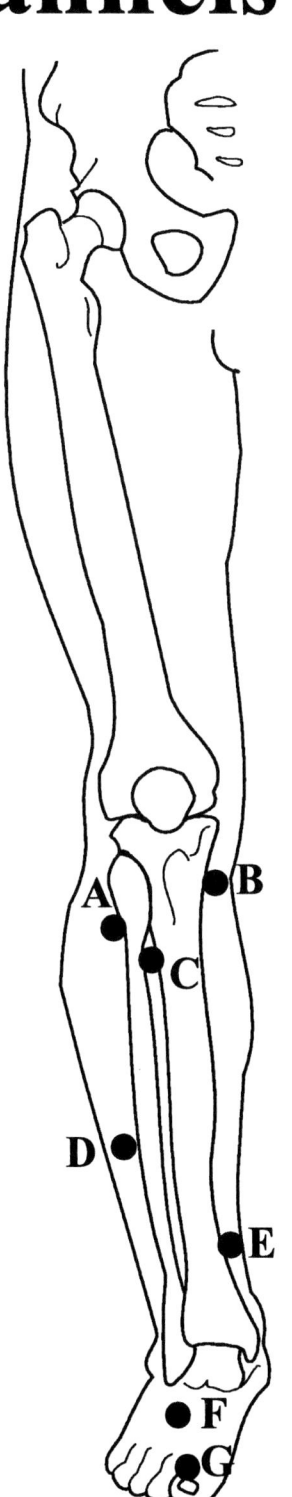

644. Which of these acupoints is the brook point on a wood channel?

    a. G

    b. F

    c. E

    d. A

Answer: _____

Source: C-221, D-474

For the following questions, refer to the diagram on the next page

645. Which of these acupoints is located in the nasolabial groove?

    a. G

    b. F

    c. E

    d. D

Answer: _____

Source: C-144, D-120

646. If acupoint C is *Shen Ting* (GV 24), and acupoint A is located about 4.5 *cun* lateral to acupoint C and is 0.5 *cun* in the hairline, what is acupoint A?

    a. *Tou Lin Qi* (GB 15)

    b. *Qu Chai* (Bl 4)

    c. *Mei Chong* (Bl 3)

    d. *Tou Wei* (St 8)

Answer: _____

Source: C-147, D-135

647. Which of these acupoints is the last point on the conception vessel?

    a. C

    b. E

    c. F

    d. G

Answer: _____

Source: C-524, D-241

648. Which of these points is on the stomach channel?

    a. B

    b. D

    c. E

    d. F

Answer: _____

Source: C-145, D-131

Sources: C=CAM, D=Deadman, F=Flaws, S=Shanghai

Mixed Channels 2

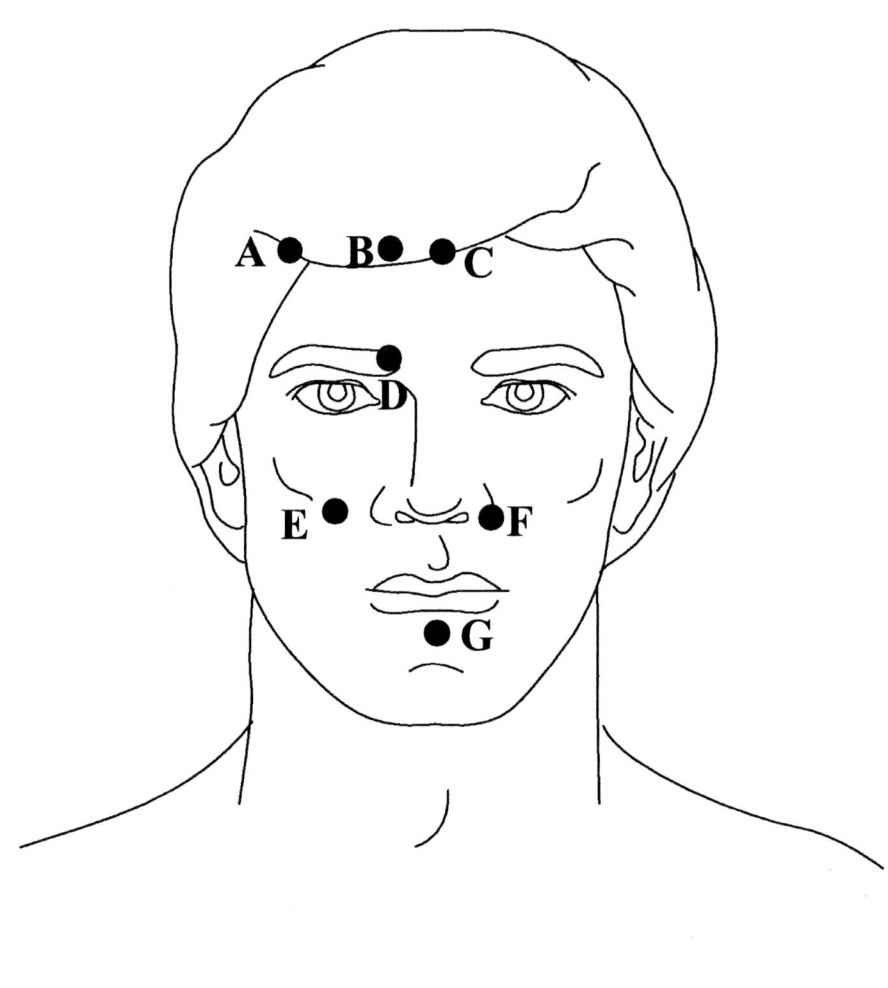

649. Acupoint B is 0.5 *cun* within the anterior hairline, and 1.5 *cun* lateral to acupoint C, which is *Shen Ting* (GV 24). Acupoint D is directly inferior to acupoint B. What is acupoint D?

    a. *Jing Ming* (Bl 1)

    b. *Zhan Zhu* (Bl 2)

    c. *Yin Tang* (M-HN-3)

    d. *Bi Tong* (M-HN-14)

Answer: _____

Source: C-174, D-257

Case Studies

Carefully read each case and then answer the questions which follow.

Case 1

A 55 year-old weekend gardener comes to see you about his back. Yesterday while lifting a hundred pound bag of fertilizer he felt a tugging in his low back and by today, he can barely stand upright. He has no sciatica or foot drag, just spasms when he stands. His pulse shows some choppiness.

650. This is a _____ pattern.

    a. Replete

    b. Vacuous

    c. Desertion

    d. Pattern

Answer: _____

Source: C-471, F-143

651. Given that the patient is in good health otherwise, what is the primary pattern that you would treat?

    a. Qi desertion

    b. Blood vacuity

    c. Qi stagnation, blood stasis

    d. Sinking of the great qi

Answer: _____

Source: C-473, F-142

652. Which non-channel point(s) would you select for this pattern?

    a. *Luo Zhen* (M-UE-24)

    b. *Yao Tong Xue* (N-UE-19)

    c. *Jian Qian* (M-UE-48)

    d. *He Ding* (M-LE-27)

Answer: _____

Source: C-250, D-579

653. What is the correct description of the location of the acupoint(s) you have chosen in the question above?

    a. Midway between the end of the anterior axillary fold and *Jian Yu* (LI 15)

    b. In the depression of the midpoint of the superior patellar border

    c. Two points on the dorsum of each hand, between the second and third, and fourth and fifth metacarpal bones

    d. On the dorsal crease of the wrist, in the depression on the radial side of the tendon of the extensor muscles of the fingers

Answer: _____

Source: C-250, D-579

654. What additional acupuncture technique(s) would you employ for this patient's symptoms?

    a. Needle *Ren Zhong* (GV 26)

    b. Cupping of the painful area

    c. Prick to bleed *Wei Zhong* (Bl 40)

    d. All of the above

Answer: _____

Source: C-473, S-654

Case 2

A 20 year-old woman comes to your office complaining about a cold of three days duration. Her temperature is 100° F, she is producing thick, yellow mucus, and has a productive cough. Her tongue has thin, yellow fur and her pulse is rapid and floating.

655. What pattern is present here?

    a. Wind cold raiding the lungs

    b. Wind heat attacking the lungs

    c. Wind dryness damaging the lungs

    d. Phlegm heat congesting the lungs

Answer: _____

Source: C-407, F-85, S-574

656. What are the treatment principles that should be followed?

    a. Course wind and scatter cold

    b. Course wind, and clear heat

    c. Course wind, moisten dryness, and stop cough

    d. Clear heat and transform phlegm

Answer: _____

Source: F-85, S-574

657. Pick the prescription which best treats the pattern:

    a. *Feng Men* (Bl 12), *Feng Chi* (Bl 20), *Lie Que* (Lu 7), *He Gu* (LI 4)

    b. *Da Zui* (GV 14), *Qu Chi* (LI 11), *Wai Guan* (TB 5), *He Gu* (LI 4)

    c. *Feng Men* (Bl 12), *San Yin Jiao* (Sp 6), *Lie Que* (Lu 7), *He Gu* (LI 4)

    d. *Fei Shu* (Bl 13), *Chi Ze* (Lu 5), *Feng Long* (St 40), *He Gu* (LI 4)

Answer: _____

Source: C-407, S-574

658. Refer to figure CS1 below and answer this question:

The source point of the large intestine channel would be an important one in the treatment of this pattern. Identify it.

    a. A

    b. D

    c. E

    d. None of the above

Answer: _____

Source: C-140, D-103

659. What needling method should be used on the points in this prescription?

    a. Draining

    b. Supplementation

    c. *Gua sha*

    d. None of the above

Answer: _____

Source: C-407, S-474

Posterior View

CS1

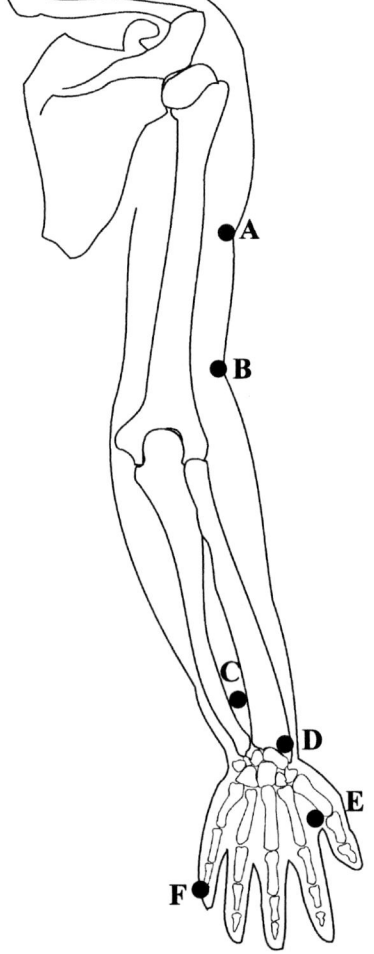

Sources: C=CAM, D=Deadman, F=Flaws, S=Shanghai

Case 3

A 36 year-old man comes to see you because he has been afflicted by boils for the last year. He has taken many rounds of antibiotics which only temporarily clear the problem. Skin washing with antibacterial soaps have little effect. He presents with several furuncles on his buttocks and two on his upper back.

660. Which acupoints on which channels should be selected to treat this problem?

    a. Foot *tai yin*, hand *yang ming*

    b. Foot *jue yin*, foot *yang ming*

    c. Hand *yang ming*, governing vessel

    d. Foot *yang ming*, conception vessel

Answer: _____

Source: C-515, S-636

661. Which acupoints should be included in your prescription?

    a. *Xue Hai* (Sp 10), *Qu Chi* (LI 11)

    b. *Tai Chong* (Liv 3), *Zu San Li* (St 36)

    c. *He Gu* (LI 4), *Ling Tai* (GV 10)

    d. *Zu San Li* (St 36), *Zhong Wan* (CV 12)

Answer: _____

Source: C-515, S-636

662. Which acupoint should be pricked to bleed to relieve the furuncles on the patient's back and legs?

    a. *Da Zhui* (GV 14)

    b. *Fei Yang* (Bl 58)

    c. *Wai Qiu* (GB 36)

    d. *Wei Zhong* (Bl 40)

Answer: _____

Source: C-515, S-636

663. What is the correct description of the location of the acupoint you have chosen in the question above?

    a. 7 *cun* directly above *Kun Lun* (Bl 60), on the posterior border of the fibula

    b. Midpoint of the transverse crease of the popliteal fossa

    c. 7 *cun* above the tip of the external malleolus on the anterior border of the fibula

    d. Below the spinous process of the 7th cervical vertebra, approximately at the level of the shoulders

Answer: _____

Source: C-184, D-299

664. If left unattended these boils can cause an inflammation of the nearby lymph system. This condition is called:

    a. Carbuncle

    b. Erysipelas

    c. Red thread boil

    d. Zoster boil

Answer: _____

Source: C-515, S-636

Case 4

A 30 year old woman arrives at your practice for the treatment of chronic yeast infections. She has applied anti-fungal creams and taken a prescription drug, but the infections keep on returning. She reports that her discharge is thick, yellow, and has a strong odor, she has an intense vulvar itch, and has had some constipation and a dry mouth the last several days. Her tongue has sticky, yellow fur and her pulse is bowstring and rapid.

665. What is the Chinese medical pattern?

     a. Spleen qi vacuity

     b. Kidney qi vacuity

     c. Damp heat in the lower burner

     d. Liver depression, spleen vacuity

Answer: _____

Source: C-493, S-675

666. What should your treatment principles be?

     a. Boost the qi and fortify the spleen

     b. Boost the qi and invigorate the kidneys

     c. Clear heat and eliminate dampness

     d. Course the liver and fortify the spleen

Answer: _____

Source: C-495, S-675

667. To address the vulvar itching, which acupoint would be most appropriate?

     a. *Li Gou* (Liv 5)

     b. *San Yin Jiao* (Sp 6)

     c. *Tai Chong* (Liv 3)

     d. *Yin Ling Quan* (Sp 9)

Answer: _____

Source: C-495, D-482

668. Refer to figure CS2 below and answer this question:

Which of these acupoints reflects the correct response to the question above?

    a. C

    b. E

    c. D

    d. None of the above

Answer: _____

Source: C-495, D-482

CS2

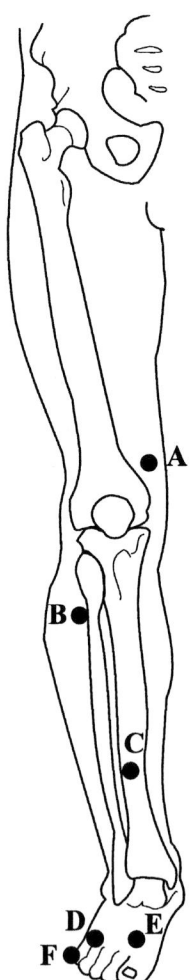

Anterior View

Sources: C=CAM, D=Deadman, F=Flaws, S=Shanghai

Case 5

A 27 year-old woman comes to see you directly from the tennis court at the insistence of her doubles partner. She reports a headache, dizziness, profuse sweating, dry mouth and tongue, and extreme thirst. Her pulse is floating, large, and rapid.

669. What is this patient experiencing?

     a. Wind stroke

     b. Summerheat (mild)

     c. Blood stasis

     d. Yin vacuity

Answer: _____

Source: C-404, S-568

670. What is the first point that should be needled and the most important one for treating this condition?

     a. *Tai Chong* (Liv 3)

     b. *Da Zhui* (GV 14)

     c. *He Gu* (LI 4)

     d. *Tai Xi* (Ki 3)

Answer: _____

Source: C-405, S-569

671. What is the correct description of the location of the acupoint you have chosen in the question above?

     a. Below the spinous process of the 7th thoracic vertebra

     b. In the depression between the tip of the medial maleolus and Achilles tendon

     c. On the dorsum of the foot, in the depression distal to the junction of the first and second metatarsal bones

     d. Between the first and second metacarpal bones, approximately in the middle of the second metacarpal bone on the radial side

Answer: _____

Source: C-405, S-569

672. If the patient had a more severe form of this condition and had fainted, which point should be added to the prescription?

      a. *Bai Hui* (GV 20)

      b. *Yong Quan* (Ki 1)

      c. *Shao Chong* (Ht 9)

      d. *Ren Zhong* (GV 26)

Answer: _____

Source: C-405, S-569

673. What point on the lower limbs is often added to quickly drain heat from a patient suffering from this condition?

      a. *San Yin Jiao* (Sp 6)

      b. *Tai Xi* (Ki 3)

      c. *Wei Zhong* (Bl 40)

      d. *Da Dun* (Liv 1)

Answer: _____

Source: C-405, S-569

Case 6

A 32 year-old man arrives at your office with severe abdominal pain in the lower right quadrant of his abdomen. The pain started last night after a rich, spicy meal. About two hours later he began vomiting. The vomiting has ceased, but this morning, he has no appetite and is running a fever of 99°F. His tongue is red with slimy, yellow fur. His pulse is slippery and rapid.

674. What is the most probable Chinese medical pattern this patient is presenting?

    a. Large intestine heat stasis

    b. Large intestine qi stagnation

    c. Large intestine damp heat

    d. Large intestine vacuity cold

Answer: _____

Source: C-517, F-117, S-639

675. In performing your examination, you note that the patient has two troubling signs. One is pain around *Tian Shu* (St 25) on the right side, the other is:

    a. Acid reflux

    b. Cold around *Zhong Wan* (St 12)

    c. Pain and inability to fully extend the right leg

    d. Local tenderness when *He Gu* (LI 4) is pressed

Answer: _____

Source: C-517

676. In continuing your examination, you note that one acupoint on the lower extremities is especially tender. Which acupoint is it?

    a. *Tai Xi* (Ki 3)

    b. *Dan Nang Xue* (M-LE-23)

    c. *Lan Wei Xue* (M-LE-13)

    d. *Tai Chong* (Liv 13)

Answer: _____

Source: C-252, D-583

677. Refer to figure CS2 below and answer this question:

Which of these acupoints reflects the correct response to the question above?

    a. A

    b. B

    c. C

    d. None of the above

Answer: _____

Source: C-495, D-482

678. You decide to treat the patient, but what should you do if he has not improved or becomes worse?

    a. Add herbs to your acupuncture prescription.

    b. Tell him to be patient, treatments often take a day or so to be effective.

    c. Refer him to his Western physician for more tests.

    d. Tell the patient to return for more aggressive treatment.

Answer: _____

Source: C-518, F-117

Anterior View

CS2

Sources: C=CAM, D=Deadman, F=Flaws, S=Shanghai

Case 7

A patient comes to see you with the Western diagnosis of "torticollis." Now answer the following questions about this patient.

679. What is wrong with the patient?

    a. Sprained back

    b. Sore ankle

    c. Twisted knee

    d. Stiff neck

Answer: _____

Source: C-521, S-661

680. Which non-channel acupoint is best for treating this problem?

    a. *Yao Tong Xue* (N-UE-19)

    b. *Ba Xie* (M-UE-22)

    c. *Er Bai* (M-UE-29)

    d. *Luo Zhen* (M-UE-24)

Answer: _____

Source: C-521, D-579, S-661

681. What is the correct description of the location of the acupoint(s) you have chosen in the question above?

    a. On the dorsum of the hand, at the junction of the red and white skin of the hand webs

    b. On the flexor aspect of the forearm, 4 *cun* proximal to *Da Ling* (Per 7)

    c. Two points on the dorsum of each hand, between the second and third, and fourth and fifth metacarpal bones

    d. On the dorsum of the hand, between the second and third metacarpal bones, 0.5 *cun* posterior to the metacarpolphalangeal joint

Answer: _____

Source: C-250, D-579, S-661

682. What is the most common cause of this problem?

    a. Heavy lifting

    b. Running on uneven ground

    c. Playing football or soccer

    d. Sleeping in an awkward position or near an open window

Answer: _____

Source: C-521, S-661

683. What is (are) the evil(s) that causes this problem?

    a. Traumatic injury

    b. Wind and heat

    c. Wind and cold

    d. Dampness

Answer: _____

Source: C-521, S-661

Case 8

A 23 year-old nursing mother comes to see you because she has begun experiencing pain in her right breast and has ceased to produce milk. Her Western physician wants to give her antibiotics, but she is afraid they will get into her milk. She says that the breast is now very swollen and has a lump in it. Her pulse is slippery and rapid.

684. What has happened to the patient?

    a. Her milk has dried up

    b. She is malnourished

    c. She has developed mastitis

    d. She is pregnant again

Answer: _____

Source: C-516, S-637

685. What evils are causing her condition?

    a. Dampness and heat

    b. Dampness and cold

    c. Qi vacuity

    d. Blood vacuity

Answer: _____

Source: C-516, S-637

686. What is the appropriate prescription for treating this condition?

    a. *Dan Zhong* (CV 17), *Shao Ze* (SI 1), *Ru Gen* (St 18)

    b. *He Gu* (LI 4), *Tai Chong* (Liv 3), *Qi Men* (Liv 14)

    c. *Qi Hai* (CV 6), *Zu San Li* (St 36), *Tai Xi* (Ki 3)

    d. *Ge Shu* (Bl 17), *Zu San Li* (St 36), *Zhong Wan* (CV 12)

Answer: _____

Source: C-516, S-637

687. To reduce the swelling and pain in the breast, what acupoint should be added to the prescription?

    a. *Ru Zhong* (St 17)

    b. *Wai Guan* (TB 5)

    c. *He Gu* (LI 4)

    d. *Zu Lin Qi* (GB 41)

Answer: _____

Source: C-517, D-460

688. Refer to figure CS2 below and answer this question:

Which of these acupoints reflects the correct response to the question above?

    a. D

    b. E

    c. F

    d. None of the above

Answer: _____

Source: C-220, D-460

Anterior View

CS2

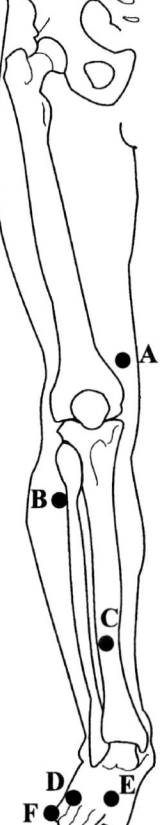

Case 9

A 61 year-old man comes to see you because he has been experiencing hearing loss. For the past year he has noticed a decline in his hearing and has had increased tinnitus. A hearing exam yielded some loss in high and low tones but not enough to qualify him for a hearing aid. In the asking examination, he notes that he has had increased low back and knee pain and that he gets up more often to urinate at night. His tongue is pale and his pulses are generally deep and weak.

689. What is the Chinese medical pattern associated with the hearing loss?

    a. Kidney yin vacuity

    b. Kidney qi vacuity

    c. Kidney not absorbing the qi

    d. Kidney vacuity, water spilling over

Answer: _____

Source: C-522, F-119, S-688

690. What acupuncture prescription would help remedy both the hearing loss and tinnitus?

    a. *Shen Shu* (Bl 23), *Tai Xi* (Ki 3), *San Yin Jiao* (Sp 6)

    b. *Shen Shu* (Bl 23), *Ming Men* (GV 4), *Yi Feng* (TB 17)

    c. *Shen Shu* (Bl 23), *Tai Xi* (Ki 3), *Fei Shu* (Bl 13)

    d. *Shen Shu* (Bl 23), *Shui Fen* (CV 9), *Yin Ling Quan* (Sp 9)

Answer: _____

Source: C-523, S-688

691. If the patient were experiencing a roaring in his ears, headache, and bitter taste in his mouth, what viscera/bowels would be involved?

    a. Spleen/stomach

    b. Liver/gallbladder

    c. Heart/small intestine

    d. Lung/large intestine

Answer: _____

Source: C-522, S-688

692. If that were the case, what acupoint would quell the roaring?

    a. *Tai Xi* (Ki 3)

    b. *Wai Qiu* (GB 36)

    c. *Xing Jian* (Liv 2)

    d. *Shen Men* (Ht 7)

Answer: _____

Source: C-522, S-688

693. Refer to figure CS2 below and answer this question:

Which of these acupoints reflects the correct response to the question above?

    a. F

    b. E

    c. D

    d. None of the above

Answer: _____

Source: C-221, D-474

Anterior View

CS2

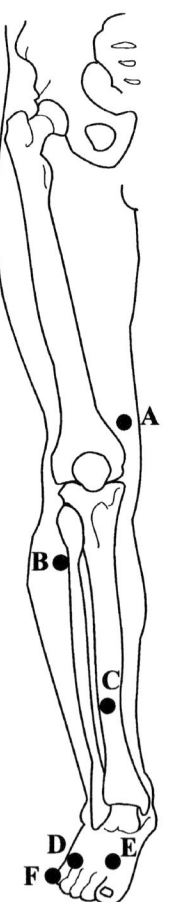

Case 10

A 42 year-old woman comes to your clinic complaining of spotting throughout her menstrual cycle. She says that her menstrual blood is light red and thin, and her menses never seem to stop. She is tired all the time, and her appetite is poor. Her tongue is pale, and her pulse is fine and forceless.

694. What is the Chinese medical pattern?

    a. Yang vacuity

    b. Qi and blood vacuity

    c. Heart/liver blood vacuity

    d. Liver depression, spleen vacuity

Answer: _____

Source: C-492, S-672

695. In addition to cutaneous needling, what technique would be most helpful for this patient in stopping her spotting?

    a. Dermabrasion

    b. Cupping

    c. Moxibustion

    d. Bleeding

Answer: _____

Source: C-492, S-672

696. To which acupoints should the technique above be applied?

    a. *Jian Jing* (GB 21)

    b. *Zu San Li* (St 36)

    c. *Zhang Men* (Liv 13)

    d. *Yin Bai* (Sp 1)

Answer: _____

Source: C-492, S-672

697. What is the correct description of the location of the acupoint you have chosen in the question above?

    a. Midway between *Da Zhui* (GV 14), and the tip of the acromion, at the crest of the trapezius muscle

    b. On the medial side of the great toe, 0.1 *cun* posterior to the corner of the nail

    c. On the lateral side of the abdomen, below the free end of the 11th rib

    d. 3 *cun* below the lower border of the patella, one finger breadth from the anterior border of the tibia

    Answer: _____

    Source: C-157, D-182

698. If this were a replete condition caused by heat, what would the menstrual blood look like?

    a. Dark purple, clotted

    b. Bright red, copious

    c. Light purplish, thin

    d. None of the above

Answer: _____

Source: C-492, S-672

Case 11

In late afternoon, a 44 year-old man comes to your office complaining that the shrimp he ate at lunch "disagreed with him." He vomited a short while ago and now his body is covered with bright red wheals. He has a slight wheeze, and his face is red. He has thin, yellow fur on his tongue, and his pulse is rapid.

699. What has happened to this patient?

    a. He is having a panic attack.

    b. He is suffering from food poisoning.

    c. He has developed allergic urticaria.

    d. He is coming down with a cold and has developed asthma.

Answer: _____

Source: C-511, S-664

700. What is the Chinese medical pattern presented here?

    a. Wind heat

    b. Wind damp

    c. Heat in the stomach and intestines, heat in the blood

    d. Fire toxins in the stomach and intestines

Answer: _____

Source: C-511, S-664

701. What treatment principles should be applied?

    a. Dispel wind and clear heat

    b. Dispel wind and drain damp

    c. Clear heat from the stomach and intestines, cool the blood

    d. Discharge fire from the stomach and intestines, and resolve toxins

Answer: _____

Source: C-511, S-664

702. Which of these acupoint prescriptions would be most appropriate?

    a. *Qu Chi* (LI 11), *He Gu* (LI 4), *Wai Guan* (TB 5), *Da Zhui* (GV 14)

    b. *Nei Guan* (Pc 6), *Zhong Wan* (CV 12), *Zu San Li* (St 36), *Shen Men* (Ht 7)

    c. *Qu Chi* (LI 11), *He Gu* (LI 4), *Xue Hai* (Sp 10), *San Yin Jiao* (Sp 6)

    d. *Lie Que* (Lu 7), *Shui Fen* (CV 9), *Yin Ling Quan* (Sp 9), *Tai Chong* (Liv 3)

Answer: _____

Source: C-511, S-664

703. A number of texts recommend a plum blossom needle on the acupoint known as the "sea of blood" to treat this condition. Refer to figure CS2 below and identify this acupoint.

    a. A

    b. B

    c. E

    d. None of the above

Answer: _____

Source: C-160, D-196

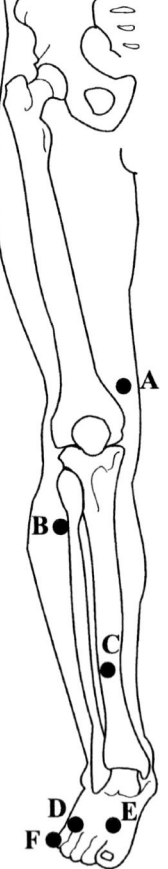

Anterior View

CS2

Case 12

A mother brings her 16 year-old daughter to see you because she has suddenly stopped menstruating. The girl experienced menarche two years ago and, despite having occasional dysmenorrhea with dark, clotted blood, has had normal cycles. She currently is having a hard time at school and cries easily. Her tongue is normal, but her pulse is bowstring and choppy.

704. What Chinese medical blood pattern is illustrated by the patient's sudden cease of menses?

    a. Qi and blood vacuity

    b. Blood stasis

    c. Heat in the blood

    d. Blood desertion

Answer: _____

Source: C-488, S-669

705. What is the root pattern that has caused the menses to cease?

    a. Spleen qi vacuity

    b. Heart/liver blood vacuity

    c. Liver depression, qi stagnation

    d. Kidney yang vacuity

Answer: _____

Source: C-488, F-148, S-669

706. What treatment principles should be applied to restart the patient's menses?

    a. Quicken the blood and dispel stasis

    b. Clear heat and cool the blood

    c. Nourish and regulate the blood

    d. Supplement the qi and warm the menses

Answer: _____

Source: C-488, F-148, S-669

707. Which of these acupoint combinations will best treat the patient's condition?

    a. *Xue Hai* (Sp 10), *Zhong Ji* (CV 4), *He Gu* (LI 4) *Tai Chong* (Liv 3)

    b. *Xue Hai* (Sp 10), *Qu Chi* (LI 11), *He Gu* (LI 4), *Zu San LI* (St 36)

    c. *Xue Hai* (Sp 10), *Ge Shu* (GV 17), *He Gu* (LI 4), *Zu San Li* (St 36)

    d. *Zu San Li* (St 36), *San Yin Jiao* (Sp 6), *Ge Shu* (GV 17), *Shen Shu* (Bl 23)

Answer: _____

Source: C-488, F-148, S-669

708. A key acupoint for treating this condition is the earth point on the foot *jue yin* channel. Refer to figure CS2 below and identify this acupoint.

    a. D

    b. E

    c. F

    d. None of the above

Answer: _____

Source: C-222, D-477

Anterior View

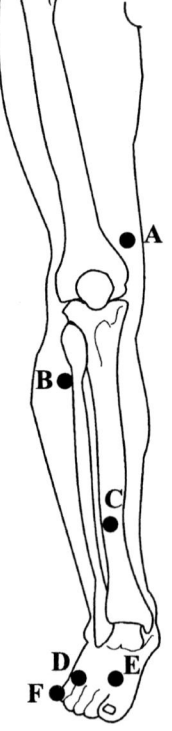

CS2

Case 13

A 38 year-old man comes to your office complaining of persistent rhinitis. His nose just used to run in the early spring and fall, but now he has problems year round. His nasal discharge today is thin and clear, and he feels well otherwise. But he says that several times a year the mucus becomes sticky and yellow, can be quite malodorous, and he will run a fever. His pulse is floating with normal speed, and his tongue has thin, white fur.

709. What is the Chinese medical pattern exhibited here?

    a. Wind cold

    b. Wind heat

    c. Wind damp

    d. Phlegm heat

Answer: _____

Source: C-524, S-689

710. Which channels should be selected for treating this patient's condition?

    a. Hand *tai yin*, foot *yang ming*

    b. Foot *tai yin*, hand *yang ming*

    c. Hand *tai yin*, hand *yang ming*

    d. Hand *yang ming*, foot *yang ming*

Answer: _____

Source: C-524, S-689

711. Which acupoint prescription would be appropriate for treating this patient today?

    a. *Lie Que* (Lu 7), *Qu Chi* (LI 11), *Wai Guan* (TB 5), *Ying Xiang* (LI 20)

    b. *Lie Que* (Lu 7), *He Gu* (LI 4), *Ying Xiang* (LI 20), *Fei Shu* (Bl 20)

    c. *Chi Ze* (Lu 5), *He Gu* (LI 4), *Tai Chong* (Liv 3), *Ying Xiang* (LI 20)

    d. *Chi Ze* (Lu 5), *Feng Long* (St 40), *Zu San Li* (St 36), *Zhong Wan* (CV 12)

Answer: _____

Source: C-524, S-689

712. A number of texts say that the network point on the hand *tai yin* channel is useful for treating this condition. Refer to figure CS1 below and identify this acupoint.

   a. C

   b. D

   c. E

   d. None of the above

Answer: _____

Source: C-138, D-83

713. Which two non-channel points would be appropriate to add to the prescription for this condition?

   a. *Yu Yao* (M-HN-6), *Tai Yang* (M-HN-9)

   b. *Er Jian* (M-HN-10), *Qiu Hou* (M-HN-8)

   c. *Yin Tang* (M-HN-3), *Bi Tong* (M-HN-14)

   d. *Jian Ming* (N-HN-3), *Ting Min* (M-HN-11)

Answer: _____

Source: C-524, S-689

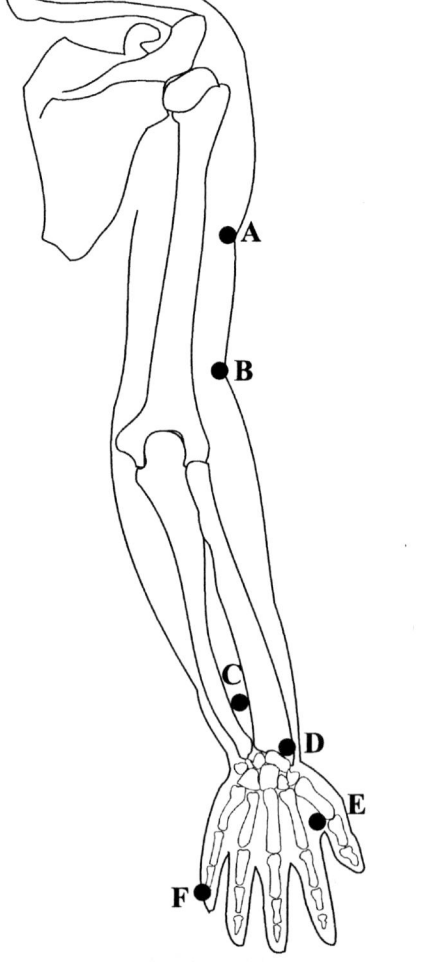

Posterior View

CS1

Case 14

A 22 year-old man comes in on a Monday after a weekend of snowboarding. Late Sunday, after his last run, he noticed that the left side of his face felt numb. Today after he woke up, the left side of his face was paralyzed, and he is now unable to close his left eye. His pulse is superficial and tight, and his tongue is pale red with thin, white fur.

714. What is the Chinese medical pattern?

      a. Qi stagnation and blood stasis

      b. Wind damp striking the channels and network vessels

      c. Wind and cold striking the channels and network vessels

      d. Blood and qi vacuity

Answer: _____

Source: C-468, F-169, S-609

715. What are the treatment principles that should be applied?

      a. Rectify the qi, and dispel stasis

      b. Dispel wind, eliminate dampness, and free the flow of the channels

      c. Dispel wind, dissipate cold, and free the flow of the channels

      d. Supplement the blood and qi

Answer: _____

Source: C-468, F-169, S-609

716. Which three channels should be needled to treat this condition?

      a. The hand and foot *yang ming*, the foot *shao yang*

      b. The hand and foot *tai yin*, the foot *yang ming*

      c. The hand and foot *jue yin*, the hand *shao yang*

      d. The hand and foot *shao yin*, the hand *yang ming*

Answer: _____

Source: C-468, S-609

717. Which of these treatments would be most appropriate for this patient?

    a. *Lie Que* (Lu 7), *He Gu* (LI 4), *Zu San Li* (St 36), *Yang Ling Quan* (GB 34)

    b. *Hou Xi* (SI 3), *He Gu* (LI 4), *Qu Chi* (LI 11), *Wai Guan* (TB 5)

    c. *Yang Bai* (GB 14), *He Gu* (LI 4), *Si Bai* (St 2), *Tong Zi Liao* (GB 1)

    d. *Nei Guan* (Per 6), *He Gu* (LI 4), *Shen Men* (Ht 7), *Tai Xi* (Ki 3)

Answer: _____

Source: C-468, S-609

718. A number of texts recommend adding *Zan Zhu* (Bl 2) for incomplete closing of the eye. What is the correct description of the location of this acupoint?

    a. In the depression slightly above the inner canthus of the eye

    b. On the medial extremity of the eyebrow, or on the supraorbital notch

    c. 0.5 *cun* lateral to the outer canthus, in the depression on the lateral side of the orbit

    d. At the midpoint of the eyebrow, directly above the pupil

Answer: _____

Source: C-174, D-257

Case 15

A new mother, age 24, comes to see you for help with her inability to nurse. She had a very difficult pregnancy and delivery, with months of morning sickness and severe hemorrhaging at birth. She was able to nurse briefly after the delivery, but her milk supply is now inadequate for the baby's needs. She is pale, as is her tongue. Her pulse is fine and forceless.

719. What has caused the inability to nurse?

    a. Stress and anguish over the pregnancy and delivery

    b. A depletion of fluids due to the morning sickness and bleeding at birth.

    c. The mother isn't trying hard enough.

    d. The mother has some sort of wind evils blocking the flow of milk.

Answer: _____

Source: C-499, S-677

720. What is the Chinese medical pattern that this patient presents?

    a. Qi stagnation and blood vacuity

    b. Liver depression, qi stagnation

    c. Qi and blood vacuity

    d. Wind cold invading the breast

Answer: _____

Source: C-499, S-677

721. What treatment principles would best remedy this problem?

    a. Regulate the qi, and supplement the blood

    b. Course the liver and rectify the qi

    c. Supplement the qi, and nourish the blood

    d. Dispel wind and cold from the breast

Answer: _____

Source: C-499, S-677

722. For all cases of insufficient lactation, both *Ru Gen* (St 18) and *Tan Zhong* (CV 17) are indicated. What three additional acupoints should be added to this prescription in this case?

      a. *Qi Men* (Liv 14), *Nei Guan* (Pc 6), *Tai Chong* (Liv 3)

      b. *Xue Hai* (Sp 10), *Zu San Li* (St 36), *Ge Shu* (Bl 17)

      c. *Pi Shu* (Bl 20), *Zu San Li* (St 36), *San Yin Jiao* (Sp 6)

      d. *Lie Que* (Lu 7), *He Gu* (LI 4), *Fei Shu* (Bl 13)

Answer: _____

Source: C-499, S-677

723. In addition to the acupoints listed above, one empirical point located on the hand is often prescribed. Refer to figure CS1 below and identify this acupoint.

      a. C

      b. D

      c. F

      d. None of the above

Answer: _____

Source: C-167, D-231

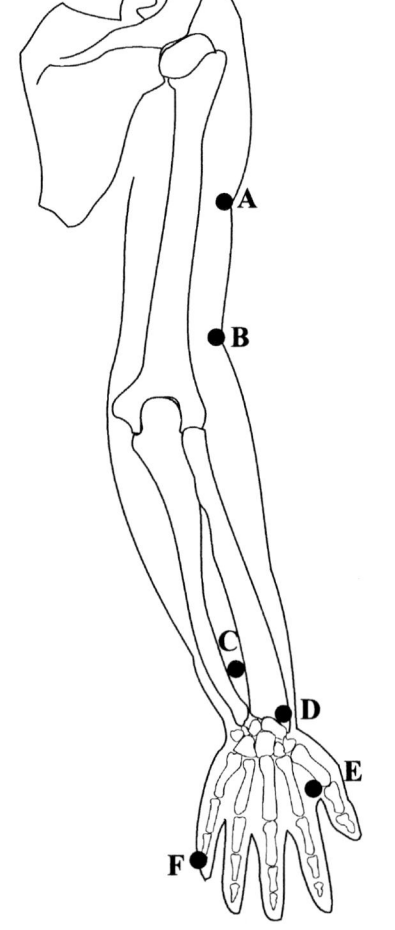

Posterior View

CS1

Sources: C=CAM, D=Deadman, F=Flaws, S=Shanghai

Case 16

A patient comes to see you in agony because he is suffering from severe diarrhea. The illness began after he had eaten some questionable food while travelling abroad in a tropical country. Since his return, he has experienced diarrhea with severe tenesmus, and his anus burns after each discharge of stool. The stool itself is thick, full of mucus, and occasionally bloody. His tongue has sticky, yellow fur, and his pulse is slippery.

724. What Chinese medical pattern presents itself here?

    a. Intestinal vacuity not securing

    b. Large intestine damp heat

    c. Large intestine vacuity cold

    d. Large intestine heat stasis

Answer: _____

Source: C-427, F-111, S-577

725. What is the cause of this condition?

    a. Hot, spicy food

    b. Unclean, poorly cooked food

    c. Sweet or fatty food

    d. All of the above

Answer: _____

Source: C-427, S-577

726. Which are the two primary acupoints used to treat this condition?

    a. *Tian Shu* (St 25), *San Yin Jiao* (Sp 6)

    b. *Zu San Li* (St 36), *Zhong Wan* (CV 12)

    c. *Tian Shu* (St 25), *Shang Ju Xu* (St 37)

    d. *Qi Hai* (CV 6), *Yin Ling Quan* (Sp 9)

Answer: _____

Source: C-427, S-577

727. What acupoint should be added to the above prescription to control the tenesmus?

    a. *Yang Ling Quan* (GB 34)

    b. *Qu Chi* (LI 11)

    c. *He Gu* (LI 4)

    d. *Zhong Lu Shu* (Bl 29)

Answer: _____

Source: C-427, D-291

728. Most texts emphasize the use of the lower uniting point of the large intestine to treat this condition. What is the correct description of the location of this acupoint?

    a. 3 *cun* below *Du Bi* (St 35), one finger-breadth from the anterior border of the tibia

    b. 6 *cun* below *Du Bi* (St 35), one finger-breadth from the anterior border of the tibia

    c. 9 *cun* below *Du Bi* (St 35), one finger-breadth from the anterior border of the tibia

    d. 8 *cun* superior to the tip of the external malleolus, two finger-breadths lateral to the anterior border of the tibia

Answer: _____

Source: C-154, D-162

Case 17

A 28 year-old, multiparous woman in the third trimester of her pregnancy comes to your clinic. She is in her thirty-third week and the child is presenting in the breech position. She has otherwise had an uneventful pregnancy and wants to try a "natural" technique before having the child forcefully turned.

729. What acumoxa technique should be used to help turn the fetus?

    a. Strong needling of *He Gu* (LI 4)

    b. Moxa cones on *Zhi Yin* (Bl 67)

    c. Seven star needling of *San Yin Jiao* (Sp 6)

    d. *Gua sha* along the eight *liao* points (Bl 31-34)

Answer: _____

Source: C-498, S-677

730. Refer to figure CS2 at the end of this section and identify the acupoint you have chosen in the question above.

    a. A

    b. D

    c. F

    d. None of the above

Answer: _____

Source: C-191, D-325

731. The technique above goes well and the child is turned to the crown position. But after the pregnancy reaches the thirty-seventh week, labor has not started. So the patient returns to ask your help in inducing labor. What acupoint(s) should be in your prescription?

    a. The eight *liao*'s (Bl 31-34)

    b. *San Yin Jiao* (Sp 6)

    c. *He Gu* (LI 4)

    d. All of the above

Answer: _____

Source: C-498, S-677

Anterior View

CS2

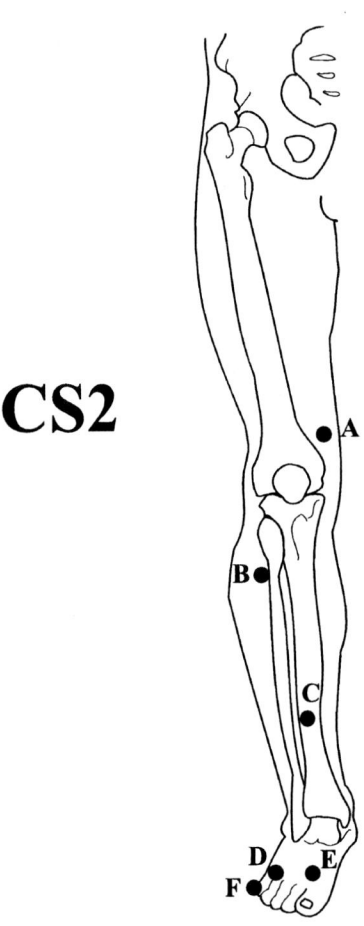

Case 18

An 20 year-old man comes to see you for frequent episodes of epistaxis. He is a large college student, and he has a very ruddy complexion. He admits that he is "a party animal" and tends to get these nosebleeds after weekends of overindulging. His tongue is red with yellow fur, and his pulse is surging.

732. What is the cause of the nosebleeds?

    a. Stress at school

    b. Diet and lifestyle

    c. Congenital weakness of the kidneys

    d. Trauma

Answer: _____

Source: C-525, F-78

733. What is the Chinese medical pattern manifested by the nosebleeds?

    a. Replete heat in the large intestines transferring to the lung

    b. Replete heat in the stomach transferring to the lung

    c. Vacuity heat in the kidney transferring to the lung

    d. Spleen qi vacuity unable to contain the blood

Answer: _____

Source: C-525, F-78

734. What acupuncture prescription would be most appropriate for this patient?

    a. *Ying Xiang* (LI 20), *He Gu* (LI 4), *Shang Xing* (GV 23)

    b. *Pi Shu* (Bl 20), *Tai Bai* (Sp 3), *Zhong Wan* (CV 12)

    c. *Shen Shu* (Bl 23), *Tai Xi* (Ki 3), *Zhao Hai* (Ki 6)

    d. *Ge Shu* (Bl 17), *Xue Hai* (Sp 10), *Zhong Kui* (Lu 6)

Answer: _____

Source: C-525, F-78

735. What acupoint on the stomach channel could be added to the prescription to clear the heat accumulated due to the overindulgence of alcohol?

    a. *Tian Shu* (St 25)

    b. *Zu San Li* (St 36)

    c. *Jie Xi* (St 41)

    d. *Nei Ting* (St 44)

Answer: _____

Source: C-525, F-78

736. What is the correct description of the location of the acupoint you have chosen in the question above?

    a. 2 *cun* lateral to the center of the umbilicus

    b. On the dorsum of the foot, at the midpoint of the transverse crease of the ankle joint

    c. 3 *cun* below *Du Bi* (St 35), one finger-breadth from the anterior border of the tibia

    d. On the dorsum of the foot, between the second and third toes, proximal to the margin of the web

Answer: _____

Source: C-156, D-171

Case 19

A 47 year-old woman comes to see you because of an embarassing problem she is having. Most days right after lunch she is afflicted with a severe case of hiccups. Her lunches are hurried affairs due to her high stress job. She says that the hiccups are loud and often accompanied by belching. Antacids help temporarily, but the hiccups return the next day. Her pulse is rapid, and her tongue is red.

737. What is the Chinese medical pattern manifested by this patient?

    a. Spleen qi vacuity

    b. Stomach qi counterflowing upward

    c. Stomach blood stasis

    d. Stomach yin vacuity

Answer: _____

Source: C-420, F-77, S-618

738. What acupuncture prescription would be most appropriate for this patient?

    a. *Pi Shu* (Sp 20), *Wei Shu* (Bl 21), *Zu San Li* (St 36), *Zhong Wan* (CV 12)

    b. *Nei Guan* (Pc 6), *Zu San Li* (St 36), *Zhong Wan* (CV 12), *Ge Shu* (Bl 17)

    c. *He Gu* (LI 4), *Zu San Li* (St 36), *Zhong Wan* (CV 12), *Xue Hai* (Sp 10)

    d. *Tai Xi* (Ki 3), *San Yin Jiao* (Sp 6), *Nei Ting* (St 44), *He Gu* (LI 4)

Answer: _____

Source: C-420, F-77, S-618

Case 20

A 72 year-old man comes to your clinic to see about his "rheumatiz." He is a rancher who spends his days exposed to the elements. His chief complaint involves his knee, which swells and becomes stiff when a weather front comes through but is especially bad when snow or rain falls. His tongue has white fur, and his pulse is bowstring.

739. What is the Chinese medical pattern manifested by this patient's condition?

   a. Moving impediment

   b. Heat impediment

   c. Wind damp impediment

   d. Cold impediment

Answer: _____

Source: C-474, F-172, S-606

740. What treatment principles should be applied?

   a. Dispel wind and clear heat

   b. Dispel wind and eliminate dampness

   c. Dispel cold

   d. Eliminate dampness and clear heat

Answer: _____

Source: C-474, F-172, S-606

741. What would be the best prescription for this patient?

   a. *Wai Guan* (TB 5), *He Gu* (LI 4), *Yin Ling Quan* (Sp 9), *Du Bi* (St 35)

   b. *Wai Guan* (TB 5), *Qu Chi* (LI 11), *Yang Ling Quan* (GB 34), *Zhi Gou* (TB 6)

   c. *Pi Shu* (Bl 20), *Yin Ling Quan* (Sp 9), *San Yin Jiao* (Sp 6), *Shui Quan* (Ki 5)

   d. *Da Zhui* (GV 14), *Shen Que* (CV 8), *Ming Men* (GV 4), *Yang Chi* (TB 4)

Answer: _____

Source: C-474, F-172, S-606

742. A key acupoint for resolving this condition is the network point on the hand *shao yang* channel. Refer to figure CS1 below and identify this acupoint.   .

    a. C

    b. D

    c. F

    d. None of the above

Answer: _____

Source: C-203, D-396

743. If the pain travelled and lodged in other joints as well as the knee, what other symptoms might occur?

    a. Sharp, stabbing pain

    b. Chills, perhaps fever

    c. Degeneration of the joints

    d. Hot, swollen joints

Answer: _____

Source: C-474, F-172, S-606

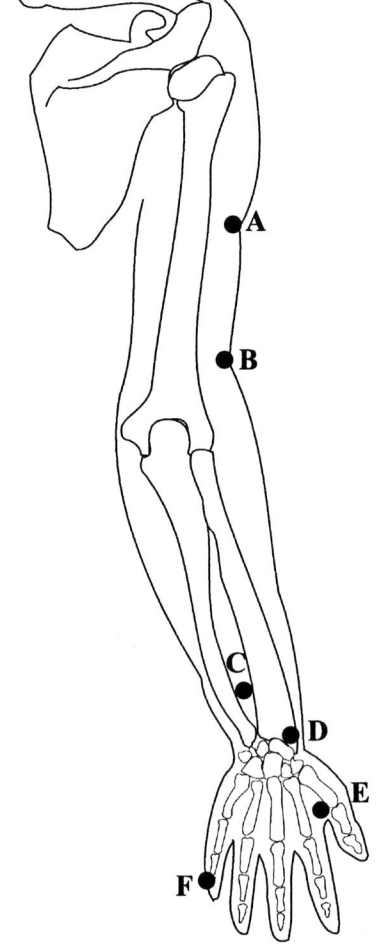

Posterior View

CS1

Case 21

A 20 year-old woman comes to your office complaining of "the period from Hell." Ever since menarche at age 13, she says that she has had very painful menses, so much so that she often has been bedridden with them. Today she complains of intense pain radiating to the sacral area. Application of a heating pad to her back and hot baths have helped ameliorate her symptoms, as have birth control pills which she now has to discontinue because of side effects. Her pulse is bowstring and the menstruate is dark purple with many clots in it.

744. What is the Chinese medical pattern illustrated here?

    a. Qi and blood vacuity

    b. Qi stagnation and blood stasis

    c. Heat in the uterus

    d. Cold in the uterus

Answer: _____

Source: C-486, F-9, S-671

745. What are the appropriate treatment principles for this patient?

    a. Supplement qi and blood

    b. Course the liver and rectify the qi, quicken the blood and dispel stasis

    c. Clear heat from the uterus

    d. Warm the uterus and regulate the menses

Answer: _____

Source: C-486, F-9, S-671

746. What is the signature pair of acupoints for treating this condition?

    a. *He Gu* (LI 4), *Tai Chong* (Liv 3)

    b. *Zu San Li* (St 36), *San Yin Jiao* (Sp 6)

    c. *Wai Guan* (TB 5), *Gong Sun* (Sp 4)

    d. *Nei Guan* (Per 6), *Zu Lin Qi* (GB 41)

Answer: _____

Source: C-486, F-9, S-671

747. What acupoint should be added to this prescription to treat the pain which radiates to the sacral area?

        a. *Zi Gong* (M-CA-18)

        b. *Di Ji* (Sp 8)

        c. *Ci Liao* (Bl 32)

        d. *Gui Lai* (St 29)

Answer: _____

Source: C-182, D-293

748. What is the correct description of the location of the acupoint you have chosen in the question above?

        a. 3 *cun* lateral to *Zhong Ji* (CV 3)

        b. 4 *cun* below the umbilicus, 2 *cun* lateral to *Zhong Ji* (CV 3)

        c. 3 *cun* below *Yin Ling Quan* (Sp 9) in the depression just posterior to the medial crest of the tibia

        d. Over the second posterior sacral foramen

Answer: _____

Source: C-182, D-293

Case 22

A 35 year old man visits you complaining of frequent headaches. These headaches became worse in the past year as his job as a stock broker became more frustrating. The headaches are one-sided, confined to the temporal area, and are always preceded by "wavy lines" in his visual field. When the pain strikes, he says he is incapacitated for hours due to severe vomiting. He has a red complexion and a red tongue.

749. What is the Chinese medical pattern illustrated here?

    a. Qi and blood vacuity

    b. Liver blood insufficiency engendering wind

    c. Ascendant liver yang hyperactivity

    d. Blood stasis

Answer: _____

Source: C-463, F-25

750. Based on how the patient presents and the pattern you chose above, what would be the pulse picture when the patient is suffering one of these headaches?

    a. Fine

    b. Choppy

    c. Vacuous

    d. Bowstring

Answer: _____

Source: C-463, F-26

Answer Key

1.B	45.C	89.D	133.C	177.C	221.D
2.A	46.C	90.B	134.D	178.B	222.C
3.C	47.A	91.D	135.A	179.C	223.D
4.A	48.C	92.A	136.C	180.A	224.B
5.B	49.D	93.B	137.B	181.B	225.C
6.D	50.D	94.D	138.A	182.C	226.B
7.C	51.B	95.B	139.D	183.D	227.A
8.C	52.D	96.B	140.B	184.B	228.C
9.B	53.C	97.D	141.A	185.C	229.B
10.C	54.C	98.C	142.B	186.B	230.D
11.C	55.D	99.D	143.C	187.A	231.C
12.D	56.C	100.B	144.A	188.D	232.B
13.B	57.C	101.C	145.C	189.D	233.A
14.A	58.B	102.C	146.C	190.C	234.D
15.B	59.D	103.D	147.D	191.D	235.D
16.B	60.C	104.B	148.A	192.C	236.D
17.B	61.B	105.B	149.A	193.C	237.C
18.A	62.C	106.A	150.C	194.B	238.C
19.D	63.B	107.C	151.D	195.C	239.D
20.D	64.B	108.B	152.C	196.D	240.C
21.C	65.C	109.B	153.D	197.B	241.A
22.B	66.C	110.B	154.B	198.D	242.C
23.C	67.A	111.C	155.A	199.C	243.A
24.B	68.B	112.B	156.C	200.D	244.B
25.D	69.C	113.A	157.D	201.D	245.D
26.B	70.C	114.C	158.C	202.B	246.C
27.A	71.B	115.A	159.D	203.C	247.B
28.A	72.B	116.C	160.B	204.A	248.A
29.B	73.D	117.D	161.D	205.B	249.C
30.D	74.B	118.D	162.C	206.B	250.D
31.C	75.D	119.A	163.C	207.D	251.B
32.C	76.C	120.C	164.D	208.C	252.A
33.D	77.D	121.D	165.A	209.B	253.B
34.A	78.A	122.B	166.D	210.C	254.C
35.C	79.A	123.B	167.B	211.D	255.A
36.D	80.D	124.D	168.B	212.B	256.C
37.B	81.A	125.A	169.B	213.D	257.D
38.D	82.C	126.C	170.C	214.D	258.C
39.A	83.D	127.D	171.D	215.C	259.B
40.C	84.B	128.A	172.D	216.B	260.B
41.B	85.B	129.C	173.D	217.D	261.D
42.C	86.A	130.D	174.B	218.C	262.D
43.B	87.C	131.D	175.D	219.A	263.D
44.D	88.C	132.B	176.A	220.B	264.C

265.B	*319.B	373.B	427.A	481.C	535.C
266.D	*320.A	374.A	428.B	482.B	536.B
267.C	*321.C	375.C	429.C	483.B	537.D
268.A	*322.B	376.B	430.C	484.D	538.B
269.B	*323.D	377.B	431.C	485.C	539.C
270.C	*324.B	378.D	432.C	486.B	540.C
271.D	*325.C	379.D	433.B	487.C	541.B
272.C	*326.D	380.B	434.C	488.C	542.B
273.C	*327.B	381.B	435.B	489.A	543.C
274.C	328.C	382.B	436.D	490.D	544.D
275.B	329.B	383.B	437.C	491.A	545.C
276.A	330.C	384.C	438.B	492.B	546.C
277.B	331.D	385.B	439.C	493.C	547.B
278.D	332.B	386.B	440.D	494.C	548.A
279.A	333.C	387.C	441.A	495.C	549.C
280.D	334.D	388.B	442.C	496.A	550.B
281.B	335.B	389.B	443.C	497.D	551.C
282.A	336.C	390.D	444.D	498.C	552.A
283.C	337.B	391.C	445.D	499.C	553.B
284.C	338.A	392.D	446.A	500.D	554.D
285.B	339.D	393.B	447.B	501.C	555.B
286.D	340.C	394.D	448.B	502.D	556.C
287.A	341.C	395.D	449.C	503.D	557.D
288.C	342.D	396.B	450.D	504.C	558.B
289.B	343.B	397.C	451.A	505.A	559.A
290.D	344.D	398.D	452.B	506.D	560.D
291.D	345.C	399.B	453.C	507.C	561.C
292.A	346.A	400.C	454.D	508.B	562.A
293.C	347.D	401.B	455.C	509.A	563.B
294.B	348.C	402.D	456.B	510.B	564.C
295.D	349.D	403.D	457.D	511.C	565.C
296.C	350.B	404.B	458.C	512.C	566.C
297.B	351.C	405.B	459.B	513.C	567.D
298.A	352.A	406.B	460.D	514.A	568.D
299.B	353.D	407.C	461.B	515.C	569.B
300.D	354.C	408.B	462.A	516.D	570.C
301.C	355.B	409.D	463.C	517.B	571.A
302.B	356.C	410.B	464.D	518.D	572.B
303.A	357.B	411.D	465.D	519.C	573.C
304.D	358.A	412.A	466.C	520.B	574.A
305.C	359.B	413.B	467.D	521.D	575.C
306.C	360.C	414.C	468.C	522.C	576.D
307.B	361.D	415.C	469.B	523.D	577.C
308.C	362.C	416.C	470.B	524.A	578.C
309.D	363.A	417.A	471.C	525.D	579.C
310.B	364.B	418.B	472.D	526.D	580.A
311.A	365.C	419.C	473.C	527.B	581.C
312.B	366.D	420.C	474.C	528.B	582.D
313.C	367.D	421.C	475.B	529.D	583.B
314.D	368.C	422.D	476.B	530.C	584.C
315.B	369.B	423.B	477.D	531.A	585.D
316.C	370.A	424.C	478.A	532.B	586.B
317.A	371.C	425.C	479.D	533.B	587.B
*318.C	372.B	426.A	480.D	534.D	588.C

589.A	616.C	643.C	670.B	697.B	724.B
590.C	617.A	644.A	671.A	698.B	725.D
591.B	618.C	645.B	672.D	699.C	726.C
592.C	619.D	646.D	673.C	700.C	727.D
593.C	620.B	647.D	674.A	701.C	728.B
594.B	621.C	648.C	675.C	702.C	729.B
595.A	622.B	649.B	676.C	703.A	730.C
596.C	623.A	650.A	677.B	704.B	731.D
597.B	624.B	651.C	678.C	705.C	732.B
598.C	625.B	652.B	679.D	706.A	733.B
599.B	626.A	653.C	680.D	707.A	734.A
600.D	627.C	654.D	681.D	708.B	735.D
601.C	628.D	655.B	682.D	709.A	736.D
602.D	629.B	656.B	683.C	710.C	737.B
603.B	630.A	657.B	684.C	711.B	738.B
604.B	631.C	658.C	685.A	712.D	739.C
605.A	632.B	659.A	686.A	713.C	740.B
606.C	633.D	660.C	687.D	714.C	741.A
607.D	634.B	661.C	688.A	715.C	742.A
608.A	635.C	662.D	689.B	716.A	743.B
609.B	636.D	663.B	690.B	717.C	744.B
610.B	637.A	664.C	691.B	718.B	745.B
611.D	638.D	665.C	692.C	719.B	746.A
612.C	639.B	666.C	693.D	720.C	747.C
613.C	640.B	667.A	694.B	721.C	748.D
614.B	641.B	668.A	695.C	722.C	749.C
615.D	642.C	669.B	696.D	723.C	750.D

*For each of the ten questions 318-327 you will be given the logic for the answer below:

318. Logic: *Jin Men* (Bl 63) is not a source point.

319. Logic: *Xuan Zhong* (GB 39) is not an alarm point.

320. Logic: *He Gu* (LI 4) is not the master point of an extraordinary vessel.

321. Logic: *Pian Li* (LI 6) is not a cleft point.

322. Logic: *Tai Chong* (Liv 3) is not a master point.

323. Logic: *Da Ling* (Per 7) is not a network point.

324. Logic: *Wan Gu* (SI 4) is not a stream point.

325. Logic: *Fu Liu* (Ki 7) is not a uniting point.

326. Logic: *Kun Lun* (Bl 60) is not an earth phase point.

327. Logic: *Hou Xi* (SI 3) is not a drainage point.

Glossary

As with all Blue Poppy Press publications, this book uses Nigel Wiseman and Feng Ye's standard translational terminology for all Chinese medical terms. For complete definitions, see their *A Practical Dictionary of Chinese Medicine* available from Paradigm Publications. Below is a short glossary of some of the most common technical terms used in this book for those unfamiliar with Wiseman and Feng's terminology.

Alarm point (*mu xue*): Any of a group of points on the abdomen or chest, each of which connects directly to a bowel or viscus.

Back transport point(s) (*bei shu xue*): Any of the points on the bladder channel on the back which connect directly with their corresponding viscera and bowels.

Bowel(s) (*fu*): Any of the six hollow organs which convey and conduct but do not store, *e.g.*, the gallbladder, small intestine, stomach, large intestine, urinary bladder, and triple burner.

Conception vessel (*ren mai*): One of the eight extraordinary vessels which is located on the sagittal midline of the anterior surface of the body and which is also called the sea of yin.

Command point: The four points which 'command' the body and are used to treat ailments that affect those particular regions, e.g. *zu san li* (St 36)is the ruling point of the abdomen.

Drain, drainage (*xie*): One of the two basic treatment methods of Chinese medicine. In acupuncture, a strong stimulus applied to eliminate evils from the body manifesting in repletion patterns.

Girdling vessel (*dai mai*): One of the eight extraordinary vessels which encircles the waist.

Governing vessel (*du mai*): One of the eight extraordinary vessels which is mainly located on the sagittal midline of the posterior surface of the body and which is also called the sea of yang.

Master point(s) (*hui xue*): Any of eight points located on the distal portions of the upper and lower extremities which correspond and are used to treat the eight extraordinary vessels. In this case, one particular master point treats one particular extraordinary vessel, *e.g.*, *Gong Sun* (Sp 4) corresponds to and treats the penetrating vessel.

Network (point &/or vessel) (*luo*): Either the secondary channels called the network vessels or the points on the 12 regular channels which connect one paired yin or yang channel to its corresponding yin-yang partner.

Penetrating vessel (*chong mai*): Also called the thoroughfare vessel, this is one of the eight extraordinary vessels. It is also sometimes referred to as the sea of blood.

Phase (*xing*): As in the "five phases," wood, fire, earth, metal, and water.

Replete, repletion (*shi*): Fullness or strength, the opposite of vacuity, as in evil repletion.

Sinew(s) (*jin*): Tough, stringy, elastic parts of the body; also a vein visible at the surface of the body.

Supplement, supplementation (*bu*): One of the two basic treatment methods of Chinese medicine, the opposite of drainage. It is a method of treatment derived from the principles, "vacuity is treated by supplementing," and "detriment is treated by boosting."

Transport points: Any of a series of five points below the elbows and knees on each of the twelve channels. The five points are the well, brook (spring), stream, river, and uniting (sea).

Vacuous, vacuity (*xu*): Weakness, emptiness, the opposite of repletion.

Viscus, viscera (*zang*): Any of the five solid organs which engender the qi and blood and store essence, *e.g.*, the liver, heart, spleen, lungs, and kidneys.

Yang linking vessel (*yang wei mai*): One of the eight extraordinary vessels.

Yin linking vessel (*yin wei mai*): One of the eight extraordinary vessels.

Yang springing vessel (*yang qiao mai*): One of the eight extraordinary vessels.

Yin springing vessel (*yin qiao mai*): One of the eight extraordinary vessels.

CURING FIBROMYALGIA NATURALLY WITH
CHINESE MEDICINE
by Bob Flaws
ISBN 1-891845-09-8

CURING HAY FEVER NATURALLY WITH
CHINESE MEDICINE
by Bob Flaws
ISBN 0-936185-91-0

CURING HEADACHES NATURALLY WITH
CHINESE MEDICINE
by Bob Flaws
ISBN 0-936185-95-3

CURING IBS NATURALLY WITH
CHINESE MEDICINE
by Jane Bean Oberski
ISBN 1-891845-11-X

CURING INSOMNIA NATURALLY WITH
CHINESE MEDICINE
by Bob Flaws
ISBN 0-936185-86-4

CURING PMS NATURALLY WITH
CHINESE MEDICINE
by Bob Flaws
ISBN 0-936185-85-6

THE DIVINE FARMER'S MATERIA MEDICA A
Translation of the Shen Nong Ben Cao
translation by Yang Shouz-zhong
ISBN 0-936185-96-1

DUI YAO: THE ART OF COMBINING
CHINESE HERBAL MEDICINALS
by Philippe Sionneau
ISBN 0-936185-81-3

ENDOMETRIOSIS, INFERTILITY AND
TRADITIONAL CHINESE MEDICINE:
A Laywoman's Guide
by Bob Flaws
ISBN 0-936185-14-7

THE ESSENCE OF LIU FENG-WU'S
GYNECOLOGY
by Liu Feng-wu, translated by Yang Shou-zhong
ISBN 0-936185-88-0

EXTRA TREATISES BASED ON
INVESTIGATION & INQUIRY:
A Translation of Zhu Dan-xi's Ge Zhi Yu Lun
translation by Yang Shou-zhong
ISBN 0-936185-53-8

FIRE IN THE VALLEY: TCM Diagnosis &
Treatment of Vaginal Diseases
by Bob Flaws
ISBN 0-936185-25-2

FU QING-ZHU'S GYNECOLOGY
trans. by Yang Shou-zhong and Liu Da-wei
ISBN 0-936185-35-X

FULFILLING THE ESSENCE:
A Handbook of Traditional & Contemporary
Treatments for Female Infertility
by Bob Flaws
ISBN 0-936185-48-1

GOLDEN NEEDLE WANG LE-TING: A 20th
Century Master's Approach to Acupuncture
by Yu Hui-chan and Han Fu-ru, trans. by Shuai Xue-
zhong
ISBN 0-936185-789-3

A GUIDE TO GYNECOLOGY
by Ye Heng-yin,
trans. by Bob Flaws and Shuai Xue-zhong
ISBN 1-891845-19-5

A HANDBOOK OF TCM PATTERNS
& TREATMENTS
by Bob Flaws & Daniel Finney
ISBN 0-936185-70-8

A HANDBOOK OF TRADITIONAL
CHINESE DERMATOLOGY
by Liang Jian-hui, trans. by Zhang Ting-liang & Bob
Flaws
ISBN 0-936185-07-4

A HANDBOOK OF TRADITIONAL
CHINESE GYNECOLOGY
by Zhejiang College of TCM, trans. by Zhang Ting-
liang & Bob Flaws
ISBN 0-936185-06-6 (4th edit.)

A HANDBOOK OF CHINESE HEMATOLOGY
by Simon Becker
ISBN 1-891845-16-0

A HANDBOOK OF MENSTRUAL DISEASES IN
CHINESE MEDICINE
by Bob Flaws
ISBN 0-936185-82-1

A HANDBOOK of TCM PEDIATRICS
by Bob Flaws
ISBN 0-936185-72-4

TEACH YOURSELF TO READ MODERN
MEDICAL CHINESE
by Bob Flaws
ISBN 0-936185-99-6

TREATING PEDIATRIC BED-WETTING WITH
ACUPUNCTURE & CHINESE MEDICINE
by Robert Helmer
ISBN 978-1-891845-33-0

THE TREATMENT OF CARDIOVASCULAR
DISEASES WITH CHINESE MEDICINE
by Simon Becker, Bob Flaws &
Robert Casañas, MD
ISBN 978-1-891845-27-6

THE TREATMENT OF DIABETES
MELLITUS WITH CHINESE MEDICINE
by Bob Flaws, Lynn Kuchinski &
Robert Casañas, M.D.
ISBN 1-891845-21-7

THE TREATMENT OF DISEASE IN TCM, Vol. 1:
Diseases of the Head & Face, Including Mental
& Emotional Disorders
by Philippe Sionneau & Lü Gang
ISBN 0-936185-69-4

THE TREATMENT OF DISEASE IN TCM, Vol. II:
Diseases of the Eyes, Ears, Nose, & Throat
by Sionneau & Lü
ISBN 0-936185-69-4

THE TREATMENT OF DISEASE, Vol. III:
Diseases of the Mouth, Lips, Tongue,
Teeth & Gums
by Sionneau & Lü
ISBN 0-936185-79-1

THE TREATMENT OF DISEASE, Vol IV:
Diseases of the Neck, Shoulders,
Back, & Limbs
by Philippe Sionneau & Lü Gang
ISBN 0-936185-89-9

THE TREATMENT OF DISEASE, Vol V: Diseases
of the Chest & Abdomen
by Philippe Sionneau & Lü Gang
ISBN 1-891845-02-0

THE TREATMENT OF DISEASE, Vol VI:
Diseases of the Urogential System
& Proctology
by Philippe Sionneau & Lü Gang
ISBN 1-891845-05-5

THE TREATMENT OF DISEASE, Vol VII:
General Symptoms
by Philippe Sionneau & Lü Gang
ISBN 1-891845-14-4

THE TREATMENT OF EXTERNAL
DISEASES WITH ACUPUNCTURE
& MOXIBUSTION
by Yan Cui-lan and Zhu Yun-long, trans. by Yang
Shou-zhong
ISBN 0-936185-80-5

THE TREATMENT OF MODERN
WESTERN MEDICAL DISEASES
WITH CHINESE MEDICINE
by Bob Flaws & Philippe Sionneau
ISBN 1-891845-20-9

THE TREATMENT OF DIABETES
MELLITUS WITH CHINESE MEDICINE
by Bob Flaws, Lynn Kuchinski
& Robert Casañas, MD
ISBN 1-891845-21-7

UNDERSTANDING THE DIFFICULT PATIENT:
A Guide for Practitioners of Oriental Medicine
by Nancy Bilello, RN, L.ac.
ISBN 1-891845-32-2

70 ESSENTIAL CHINESE
HERBAL FORMULAS
by Bob Flaws
ISBN 0-936185-59-7

160 ESSENTIAL CHINESE HERBAL PATENT
MEDICINES
by Bob Flaws
ISBN 1-891945-12-8

630 QUESTIONS & ANSWERS ABOUT
CHINESE HERBAL MEDICINE:
A Workbook & Study Guide
by Bob Flaws
ISBN 1-891845-04-7

230 ESSENTIAL CHINESE MEDICINALS
by Bob Flaws
ISBN 1-891845-03-9

750 QUESTIONS & ANSWERS ABOUT
ACUPUNCTURE
Exam Preparation & Study Guide
by Fred Jennes
ISBN 1-891845-22-5